Also Available From the
American Academy of Pediatrics

Building Happier Kids: Stress-busting Tools for Parents

The CALM Baby Method: Solutions for Fussy Days and
  Sleepless Nights

Caring for Your Baby and Young Child: Birth to Age 5*

Dad to Dad: Parenting Like a Pro

Guide to Toilet Training

Heading Home With Your Newborn: From Birth to Reality

High Five Discipline: Positive Parenting for Happy, Healthy,
  Well-Behaved Kids

My Child Is Sick! Expert Advice for Managing Common
  Illnesses and Injuries

The New Baby Blueprint: Caring for You and Your Little One

New Mother's Guide to Breastfeeding

Raising an Organized Child: 5 Steps to Boost Independence,
  Ease Frustration, and Promote Confidence

Raising Twins: Parenting Multiples From Pregnancy Through
  the School Years

Retro Baby: Timeless Activities to Boost Development—
  Without All the Gear!

Retro Toddler: More Than 100 Old-School Activities to Boost
  Development

Return to You: A Postpartum Plan for New Moms

The Working Mom Blueprint: Winning at Parenting Without
  Losing Yourself

Your Baby's First Year*

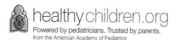

healthychildren.org
Powered by pediatricians. Trusted by parents.
from the American Academy of Pediatrics

For additional parenting resources, visit the HealthyChildren bookstore at
https://shop.aap.org/for-parents.

*This book is also available in Spanish.

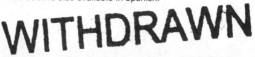
WITHDRAWN

Baby & Toddler Basics 2nd Edition

Expert Answers to Parents' Top 150 Questions

Tanya Altmann, MD, FAAP

American Academy of Pediatrics
DEDICATED TO THE HEALTH OF ALL CHILDREN®

American Academy of Pediatrics Publishing Staff

Mary Lou White, *Chief Product and Services Officer/SVP, Membership, Marketing, and Publishing*

Mark Grimes, *Vice President, Publishing*

Holly Kaminski, *Editor, Consumer Publishing*

Shannan Martin, *Production Manager, Consumer Publications*

Sara Hoerdeman, *Marketing Manager, Consumer Products*

Published by the American Academy of Pediatrics
345 Park Blvd
Itasca, IL 60143
Telephone: 630/626-6000
Facsimile: 847/434-8000
www.aap.org

The American Academy of Pediatrics is an organization of 67,000 primary care pediatricians, pediatric medical subspecialists, and pediatric surgical specialists dedicated to the health, safety, and well-being of all infants, children, adolescents, and young adults.

Printed in the United States of America
9-483/0922   1 2 3 4 5 6 7 8 9 10
CB0132
ISBN: 978-1-61002-620-8
eBook: 978-1-61002-623-9
EPUB: 978-1-61002-621-5
Cover and publication design by Scott Rattray Design
Library of Congress Control Number: 2021921246

What People Are Saying

Altmann comfortably segues between the role of knowledgeable MD and friendly mom...New and prospective parents will find that Altmann's compact, concise primer is a valuable source of reassurance and advice.

Publishers Weekly

This is a helpful resource for new parents/grandparents. It takes a no-nonsense, factual approach to commonly asked questions.

Doody's Book Reviews

Dr. Tanya manages to make you feel like your best friend and your pediatrician have come together to write this new parent guidebook, just for you. *Baby and Toddler Basics* is engaging and essential, and I know you will return to it again and again!

Samantha Ettus, work-life expert and national best-selling author of *The Pie Life: A Guilt-Free Recipe for Success and Satisfaction*

Every question parents think of is answered in this book, with up-to-date info and Dr. Tanya's experienced wisdom and tips. It's a must-have for all new parents.

Jenn Mann, author of *SuperBaby: 12 Ways to Give Your Child a Head Start in the First 3 Years* and *The A to Z Guide to Raising Happy Confident Kids*

Whether you're a first-time parent or a seasoned veteran when it comes to kids, *Baby and Toddler Basics* is sure to teach you something new and reinforce facts you already know. In a straightforward, practical manner, experienced pediatrician and mom Dr. Tanya Altmann explains the essentials of caring for a sick or healthy young child—from dealing with fevers, aches, and injuries to the basics of eating, sleeping, peeing, and pooping. This book is a necessity for all families!

> Jennifer Shu, MD, FAAP, medical editor of
> HealthyChildren.org and coauthor of *Heading Home
> With Your Newborn: From Birth to Reality* and *Food
> Fights: Winning the Nutritional Challenges of Parenthood
> With Insight, Humor, and a Bottle of Ketchup*

Dr. Tanya answers 150 of your most common baby health questions with the expertise of a trained pediatrician and the voice of a friend who's been there. Chances are, your questions are in there—and you'll love her answers.

> David L. Hill, MD, FAAP, author of *Dad to Dad:
> Parenting Like a Pro*

Once again, Dr. Tanya Altmann has hit a home run. In her characteristically warm and reassuring style, she covers every question a parent could have about knowing and caring for her new baby. *Baby and Toddler Basics* is a must-have for every new mother's home library. It's like having a pediatrician in residence! And it is an absolutely perfect baby gift!

> Betsy Brown Braun, child development/behavior
> specialist and author of *Just Tell Me What to Say* and
> *You're Not the Boss of Me*

I want to dedicate this book to every parent
with a question about caring for their baby or toddler,
you got this!

Equity, Diversity, and Inclusion Statement
The American Academy of Pediatrics is committed
to principles of equity, diversity, and inclusion in its
publishing program. Editorial boards, author selections,
and author transitions (publication succession plans)
are designed to include diverse voices that reflect society
as a whole. Editor and author teams are encouraged
to actively seek out diverse authors and reviewers at
all stages of the editorial process. Publishing staff are
committed to promoting equity, diversity, and inclusion
in all aspects of publication writing, review,
and production.

Contents

Acknowledgments   xiii

Introduction   xvii

1 Basic Baby Care   1

2 Breastfeeding   31

3 Formula Feeding   57

4 Beyond Bottles and Breastfeeding:
Starting Solid Foods   69

5 Pooping   93

6 Stomachaches and Vomiting   107

7 Fever   119

8 Coughs, Colds, and More   135

9 Vaccines   157

10 Skin   169

11 Child Care   193

12 Ingestions, Injuries, and First Aid   205

13 Growing Up   225

14 Sleep   251

Index   265

Acknowledgments

By the time this book is in print, I'll have been a physician for more than 25 years and a parent for more than 16. And I'm the first to admit that I still learn something new every day. That's one of the reasons I love my job. I learn from my patients, their parents and caregivers, colleagues, and even members of my own family. That's a lot of people to thank, so I'll try to keep this brief and focused, but know that there are many others who have also touched my life and assisted in the information I am providing throughout this book.

Starting with the staff at the American Academy of Pediatrics (AAP), who have been my support, education, colleagues, and professional family, I thank you for suggesting that I put the culmination of my pediatric career thus far on paper as *Baby and Toddler Basics*. I want to express my appreciation to the AAP Department of Publishing, including Mark Grimes and Holly Kaminski, who played an integral role in the birth of this book.

Thank you to Michelle Shuffett, MD, for your dedication to the early years of this project and lifelong friendship. Also, thank you to my mentors and the current and past interns, residents, and pediatricians at UCLA Mattel Children's Hospital for offering exceptional advice and contributions to *Baby and Toddler Basics*. In addition, thank you to Angela Beals, who helps keep my office and patients at Calabasas Pediatrics healthy and running well 24/7. Thanks to Polly Gannon, whose invaluable advice has helped not only me but my patients to successfully breastfeed, remain calm and happy, and sleep soundly through the night.

Thank you as well to the following physicians and child health experts for their review and additions to my manuscripts:

Mara Beck, MS, CCC-SLP

Brynie Collins, MD, FAAP

David Hill, MD, FAAP

Laura Jana, MD, FAAP

Alanna Levine, MD, FAAP

Catherine Pourdavoud, MD, FAAP

Angelee Reiner, MD, FAAP

Elena Rumack, DDS, MS

Beth Saltz, MPH, RD

Nina Shapiro, MD, FAAP

Jennifer Shu, MD, FAAP

Ali Strocker, MD, FAAP

Christine Katie Thang, MD, FAAP

Last, but definitely not least, thank you to my wonderful family. Thank you Melissa and Miles Remer and Diane and Clifford Numark, who provided questions and parenting insight, as well as technical and writing support. A heartfelt thanks to my sister, Candace Remer Katz, MD, an allergist and a mom who keeps me up-to-date on asthma and allergy topics and added immensely to this book and to my life.

I owe my life and many accomplishments to my parents, Donald and Louise Remer, and my grandparents who always support me and encourage me to reach for my dreams. Thanks to Grammie, Grandma, and Nana for helping to watch, play with, and teach my boys so I could see patients and write this book.

Finally, thank you to my husband Phil, the best dad ever, who really does everything and without whom I could never do all that I do. We have 3 wonderful sons, Avrick, Collen, and Maxton, who have taught me more about pediatrics and parenting than I could ever learn at the office and who are constantly making me smile with a new adventure every day. I am proud to be their mom.

Introduction

As a pediatrician, I have been answering questions from parents for over 20 years. That's why I wrote *Baby and Toddler Basics* for parents, grandparents, and caregivers. Keep this book on your nightstand or in your baby bag so when something comes up, whether a cough, a fever, a diaper rash, or a stomachache, you'll have the answer you need in a simple, concise, accurate, and easy-to-read format.

Baby and Toddler Basics focuses on your child from birth through age 3 years and includes parents' top questions on breastfeeding, nutrition, crying, sleeping, illnesses, and child care. *Baby and Toddler Basics* is meant to answer not only the questions you have today, but those you are likely to have at 3:00 am tomorrow! *Baby and Toddler Basics* provides practical information, advice, and important tips and tells you when you need to call your pediatrician. Best of all, it fits in your baby bag! So before you pick up your smartphone to call, text, or email your pediatrician, check out *Baby and Toddler Basics* for your answer.

In pediatrics, situations change dramatically depending on the age of the child, so it's no surprise that the answers to many common questions will vary by age. Therefore, in this book, babies aged birth through 1 month are called **newborns**; babies aged 1 month through 1 year are called **infants**; and children aged 1 through 3 years are called **toddlers**. As with all advice, sometimes it's most important to call your pediatrician. For that reason, I've indicated those moments with a telephone symbol ((◻)).

The information and advice in this book apply equally to children of both sexes, except where noted. To indicate this, the use of masculine and feminine pronouns is alternated throughout the book.

I hope you find **Baby and Toddler Basics** helpful, but don't forget that you know your child best. You will undoubtedly come up with questions not addressed in this book. That's the nature of having kids! If ever you find yourself with unanswered questions, no matter how small or silly they may seem, go ahead and ask your pediatrician. And whenever you have more serious concerns—remember that no book, **Baby and Toddler Basics** included, can ever take the place of direct medical advice—never hesitate to call your pediatrician. After all, that's what we're here for—even at 3:00 am!

CHAPTER 1

Basic Baby Care

I f you're reading this book, congratulations on your pregnancy (or the arrival of your little one)! Chances are you're getting a good head start in anticipating what lies ahead with your new bundle of joy. Admittedly, some days may be more joyful, or at least more peaceful, than others. Whether you're trying to figure out why your baby is crying (is she hungry, wet, or tired?) or you're attempting to get her dressed and out the door for her first doctor's appointment (don't forget that new diaper bag), you will quickly realize that your life has now changed . . . forever.

Even though you've eagerly awaited and geared up for this wonderful addition to your life and family for the past 9 months (if not more), you are likely to find yourself still needing some guidance, now that you are going to become a parent. In the hospital, you will have lots of help from the nurses, lactation consultants, and doctors—all at your fingertips. You may still be reading all the must-have parenting books and spending many evenings on the phone

1

with your mother and friends talking about all the details. You think you are prepared. But nothing can ever completely prepare you for the crazy but exciting ride ahead. Most new parents have questions, usually lots of them! Here are some of the top questions parents have.

(If it is sleep, feeding, poop, fever, or skin-related answers you're looking for, rest assured that these very important newborn topics are covered in their own chapters.)

After Delivery

1. What happens in the delivery room?

If this is your first baby, it can definitely be an overwhelming experience. But don't worry—whether you are having a vaginal delivery or a C-section, there will be designated doctors, nurses, and other specialists around to assist you and your newborn during the delivery. There will be monitors on your belly to keep track of you and your little one throughout the whole process.

After delivery, your doctor will dry and rub your baby's back and may also use a blue bulb syringe to suction her nose if needed until there's a good cry to make sure those lungs are working. Crying is a wonderful sound after delivery because it means your baby is likely strong and healthy. These are your baby's first breaths, and crying helps the lungs expand and makes residual fluid in the mouth and airway come out, which is especially important if you had a C-section. Your baby may then be placed on your chest "skin to skin" for that first moment of precious mother-baby bonding. Your baby may even search for your nipple for her first attempt at breastfeeding.

If your doctor or nurse feels that your baby needs some extra attention, she may be brought over to a warmer (in the same room) so that they can take a closer look. This will happen either immediately after delivery or after a short period of mother-baby bonding. Either way, please let the nurses and pediatricians do their job as they are quickly trying to ensure that your baby is healthy. Their priorities will be to check that the heart is beating well and the lungs are expanding properly. A spouse, family member, or birth partner may be asked if they want to cut the umbilical cord. This is optional but simple and may be a nice moment to remember. The nurse or doctor will show him or her exactly what to do (and they may even take a photo for you if you ask). After the initial minutes of going down the checklist, the nurses may weigh and measure your baby before bringing her back to you (often bundled up with a hat for warmth).

2. Should I give my baby vitamin K and eye ointment?

Yes. The vitamin K injection is one of the most important things you can do for your baby at birth because it reduces the risk of life-threatening bleeding in the first few weeks. Vitamin K is one of the essential clotting factors in the blood. All babies are born with a low amount of vitamin K due to immature organs, such as the liver and intestines, which take a few weeks to months to mature. If the vitamin K is not replaced, it puts newborns at a high risk of experiencing serious bleeding. The injection is easily given in the thigh and recommended by the American Academy of Pediatrics (AAP).

The erythromycin eye ointment is an antibiotic that prevents a bacterial eye infection that can spread from the process of delivery. Your baby may be at low risk for an infection, but the antibiotic is harmless— and it is always better to be safe than sorry, since it can prevent eye damage and blindness.

3. How can I bond with my baby?

There are many ways you can bond with your baby. Bonding is a natural process that will happen with time. It's okay if you don't feel a strong bond right away; as long as you are attending to all of your baby's needs, she will be fine. Part of the bonding process includes your baby getting to know you, in addition to you getting to know your baby. Breastfeeding is a perfect time for this, as you learn to recognize your baby's body language and facial expressions. She will learn that you are a source of comfort, and nursing will build that trust (see chapter 2 for more tips on breastfeeding). If you are bottle-feeding, these mealtimes are just as important for bonding and building a loving relationship. All parents can have skin-to-skin contact with baby, so she will feel your warmth and get used to your smell. Touching is also important, and infant massage and bath time are great ways to calm and connect to your baby. Carrying your baby in a baby carrier or a sling across your body is also a great way to help you bond and walk around easily with your baby (see the next section on when and how to go "out and about").

Baby's Bedroom?
(Or Room Share, Don't Bed Share)

Your baby doesn't necessarily need her own bedroom right now. Actually, the AAP recommends that your baby sleep in the same room as you, but in her own safe sleep space such as a crib or bassinet. Any flat, solid surface for your baby is acceptable. Sometimes, bassinets are preferred for the first few months because they may be more mobile. Otherwise, just remember that the bassinet or crib should be "bare," which means that no toys, bumper pads, pillows, or bedding should be in your baby's crib. And always place your baby to sleep on her back! If you want to decorate the room and hang items for your baby to look at, that is great—as long they are not right next to your baby at sleep time.

4. I'm feeling a little overwhelmed and down since I had my baby. Why am I not super happy, and is this normal?

It is normal to have mood swings and "baby blues" feelings after having a baby. Up to 80% of women report having some degree of the baby blues after the birth of a child, so you're not alone. A new mom may feel a little down, tired, anxious, unable to sleep (even when baby is sleeping), not as hungry as usual, or weepy—or she may cry for no apparent reason. The exact cause is not fully understood, but it's thought to be due to hormonal changes and situational and emotional changes that cause a new mom to feel down or depressed. It's important to remember that you are not alone.

The best way to feel better is to take care of yourself. Ask your friends and family for help with your baby. Or ask them for help with the housework and cooking meals (or, if possible, hire a postpartum doula or baby nurse). Remember that it's important to eat a balanced diet, get some fresh air, keep a journal, and do something you love to do.

Other things that are known to help are

- ☐ Light to moderate exercise
- ☐ Drinking plenty of fluids
- ☐ Some experts recommend taking omega-3 fatty acid, folate, magnesium, and calcium supplements (with your doctor's permission, of course)
- ☐ Avoiding caffeine and alcohol

Lack of sleep can also put you over the edge and be hard to distinguish from baby blues or postpartum depression. I remember after 4 or 5 days without sleep, I couldn't stop crying for any reason at all! Asking for help so you can get a few hours of shut-eye can really make a difference. If after a few nights of rest, you still feel anxious, hopeless, or sad and/or you don't want to get out of bed, make sure you talk to a therapist, a counselor, or your doctor. Many experts are specially trained in helping moms with baby blues and postpartum depression. In addition, new-mom support groups or other parenting classes in your area are often helpful in finding other moms with similar feelings.

I also tell breastfeeding moms' partners that their job is to get up and change the baby's diaper in the middle of the night. Or simply handing the baby to mom for a feeding and then putting the baby back in the bassinet after feeding can help mom get a little more rest, while also feeling supported.

 If your feelings of being overwhelmed or down since the birth of your baby more than 2 weeks ago seem to linger, call your obstetrician/gynecologist or primary care physician right away. Or, if these feelings have lasted more than 2 weeks straight and don't just come and go, you need to reach out to your doctor for help. In such cases, intense therapy and possibly even medications may be needed. Don't be shy about asking your family and friends for help—the birth of a baby is a special time for everyone, and they will often be more than happy to contribute.

Out and About

5. When do I need to bring my baby in for a checkup?

In general, it's a good idea to see your pediatrician within 2 to 3 days of leaving the hospital. In decades past, longer hospital stays allowed babies to be observed for about a week after delivery. This also gave parents more time to gain some hands-on newborn experience. Nowadays, the first checkup is typically scheduled soon after discharge from the hospital (within your baby's first week) to make sure your baby is feeding, peeing, and pooping well; isn't jaundiced (see question 101, on page 170); and hasn't lost too much weight. All babies initially lose weight after they are born, and most regain their birth weight by around 1 to 2 weeks of age. This early visit is especially useful because most babies spend only 2 to 3 days, at most, in the hospital after birth. That's certainly a lot to learn in a short time. How your baby is feeding, pooping, growing, and behaving will dictate how often he needs to be seen by the doctor in the first few weeks.

Remember that after being sleep deprived for 72 hours, you may barely remember your name, let alone the questions you thought of in the middle of the night. So write them down or type them up in a note on your smartphone or baby app as you think of them. Allow plenty of time to pack up (see the following Dr. Tanya's Tip: Baby Bag Essentials), get out the door, and arrive at your appointment—it can take some time to get used to moving about with a newborn!

Dr. Tanya's Tip
Baby Bag Essentials

Babies need lots of stuff—all the time. So prepare an extra baby bag ... or two. Give one to anyone else who will be caring for your baby. That way, all the necessities will be available if an outing takes longer than expected. A well-stocked diaper bag should include the following:

☐ Five diapers (at least)

☐ Changing pad

☐ Baby wipes

☐ Diaper cream

☐ Plastic bags for dirty diapers or clothes

☐ Formula, bottle, and nipple (if formula feeding); sippy cup for an older baby

☐ Burp cloths/washcloths

☐ Bottle of water (to mix formula, to clean up messes, or for mom to drink)

☐ Snack (for mom)

☐ Change of clothing (for your baby and yourself) in a sealed bag

☐ Blanket and/or nursing cover (if you desire)

☐ Pacifier (2 if your baby uses, in case one falls on the floor)

☐ Acetaminophen (Tylenol)

☐ Hand sanitizer

☐ Sunscreen (For babies under 6 months of age, when adequate clothing and shade are not available, can apply a minimal amount of sunscreen with at least 30 SPF, in small areas.)

Continued on next page

☐ Rattle or toy

☐ List of important information—pediatrician's phone number, recent weight of baby (including the date), allergies (if any), and immunization records. Better yet, save this information in your smartphone so it's always at your fingertips.

Don't forget to restock items as they are used, so you're always ready to go anywhere, anytime!

After your hospital follow-up visit, your pediatrician may recommend that your baby come in for a weight check appointment or two, but then regular well-baby examinations for the first year are usually scheduled at 1 month, 2 months, 4 months, 6 months, 9 months, and 12 months. Of course, this schedule varies slightly from doctor to doctor. It may seem like you are always on your way to the pediatrician, but every well-baby examination is important. Your doctor will examine your baby from head to toe, check his growth, evaluate his development, look for signs of illness, and provide advice for keeping your little one healthy, happy, and safe. In addition, there may be specific tests and immunizations (see chapter 9, Vaccines) recommended, depending on your baby's age at each visit.

You can always schedule an additional appointment for your baby at any time if any specific problems or concerns arise between well-child examinations.

6. When can we take our newborn out?

Whether you're thinking of going outside, inside, or high up in the sky, a good rule of thumb is to stay away from crowds of people until your baby is 6 to 8 weeks of age, if at all possible. This is because a newborn's immune system is still maturing, which leaves her more susceptible to catching colds, as well as becoming seriously ill very quickly. Avoid any closed areas where your baby could be exposed to lots of people who may be sick, such as grocery stores, malls, movie theaters, parties, or airplanes. Especially during the winter, it's best to assume that everyone is contagious—some people may not show outward symptoms but can still spread germs! Whenever possible, don't let anyone who is obviously ill get near your baby. Try to keep young children away because they tend to be even less able to keep their hands and germs to themselves. Also, try to decrease the number of people who touch, breathe on, and cough on your baby.

In addition, do your best to make sure that everyone who will be around your baby has been vaccinated against whooping cough (Tdap/DTaP), influenza, and COVID-19 (see question 100, on page 165).

Now that you know what to avoid, going outside is totally fine. Dress your baby appropriately (see the following Dr. Tanya's Tip: Is My Baby Too Hot or Too Cold?) and go for a walk in your neighborhood or enjoy a stroll outside.

Dr. Tanya's Tip
Is My Baby Too Hot or Too Cold?

You can't really know, unless you carry around a thermometer everywhere you go (which isn't realistic or recommended)! This is because babies don't always sweat or shiver when you might expect them to, and they can't yet tell you how they feel. The general rule is that babies should wear as many layers as you are wearing. It's all right to add one more layer if it makes you (or seems to make your baby) more comfortable. It's not necessary to drastically change the thermostat in your house just because you have a newborn (since parents always ask, 69°F to 72°F is a good normal range)—just dress her appropriately. If it is a hot day and you are only wearing a T-shirt and shorts, your baby should be okay in a onesie. If it is cooler out and you need a sweater and jacket, dress your baby the same. A hat is always a good idea, if it stays on! When it's cold, babies lose body heat from their heads, and when it's hot, a hat will protect them from the sun.

7. What about taking my baby on an airplane?

Keep your baby on the ground until 6 to 8 weeks of age, if at all possible. The danger is not the airplane itself but the possible contact with individuals who are both sick and contagious (see question 6, on page 11). Otherwise, the airplane poses no risk other than potential ear discomfort. The ear tubes (aka Eustachian tubes) in babies are smaller in length and different in shape than those in adults, so pressure changes during takeoff and landing (landing more so than takeoff) can sometimes cause pain. Breastfeeding, bottle-feeding, or sucking on a pacifier is often soothing during these periods because sucking and swallowing can help equalize the pressure and decrease the pain. Wait until you are sure the plane is about to take off or start its descent so your baby doesn't fill up and stop sucking too soon. Another tip for babies older than 2 months is to give an appropriate dose of acetaminophen (Tylenol) about 30 minutes prior to takeoff and, if the flight is longer than 4 hours, again prior to landing (see the Acetaminophen [Tylenol] Dosing Chart and Ibuprofen [Motrin or Advil] Dosing Chart on pages 126 and 127). It's important to note that ibuprofen isn't approved for babies younger than 6 months of age.

Dr. Tanya's Tip

Keeping Baby Healthy

Allow older siblings to gently touch or kiss your baby's toes instead of her face or hands. This will help protect your newborn from catching any illnesses that your older ones may bring home. You can also appoint your older children to be "handwashing monitors" to make sure that all visitors wash their hands before holding the baby—and that's a doctor's order!

Crying

8. My baby won't stop crying—I can't take it anymore! Is all this crying (and my frustration) normal?

Babies do cry. It's their way of communicating. Don't take it personally. He may be hungry, gassy, wet, cold, hungry, or just want to be held. The first few weeks, if he's not hungry, gas may be the culprit. You can do "gas exercises" (such as leg pumps or bicycling legs while the baby is on his back) before feeding or when your baby seems gassy or fussy. Also a little tummy time a couple of hours a day not only helps strengthen muscles but helps baby to move gas and stool, which can help reduce crying. Once your baby turns 3 months of age, you will have gotten to know him better, and you may learn to distinguish his cries and what they mean. Once a baby has been fed, burped, changed, and checked to make sure nothing is hurting him, it's generally okay to let him cry for a little while.

If your baby is crying for more than 3 hours a day, more than 3 days a week, for longer than 3 weeks, then he may have colic. Although we don't know definitively what causes colic, there are a few popular theories, and it may even be a combination of things.

One theory is that it may be related to an infant's inability to self-console because of his immature nervous system, which will improve as he gets older (usually 3–4 months). One practical approach to calming crying babies was developed by Harvey Karp, MD, FAAP. He advocates the "5 *S*'s": swaddling, side/stomach positioning while awake, shushing, swinging, and sucking. Another *S* I like to add is singing a song (your baby won't care if you can't carry a tune). Some babies also enjoy moving around, so hold your baby, dance, go for a walk, or put him in a swing. It may help both of you.

Another theory is that colic is related to newborn gut deficiency or a lack of good gut bacteria and overgrowth of unhealthy gut bacteria. The unhealthy gut bacteria cause inflammation and symptoms such as colic. By supplementing with specific strains of probiotics or good gut bacteria, you can crowd out and reduce the bad gut bacteria. Research is still underway but ask your pediatrician about starting your baby on an infant-specific probiotic to see if that can help decrease colic symptoms.

 Call your pediatrician if your baby has high-pitched or excessive crying or is truly inconsolable (the crying won't stop no matter what you do) because severe crying can be a sign of illness.

9. What's the best way to swaddle my baby and for how long?

Swaddling is the art of wrapping your baby like a burrito to help calm her and promote sleep. New parents often learn how to swaddle their baby from the nurses in the hospital. There are a few techniques, but here are the step-by-step instructions for a common swaddle. Make sure there is plenty of room around baby's hips.

Place a blanket on a flat surface, with one corner facing you (so it looks like a diamond), and fold down the top corner of the diamond by several inches. Lay your baby down with her shoulders flush with the folded-down edge. Then take either the right or left corner of the blanket and pull it across your baby's body, making sure that the arm on that side is tucked in a comfortable flexed position (bent at the elbow and placed down at her side or in front). Tightly tuck in the corner of the blanket underneath her bottom. Next, bring the bottom corner up toward the center (your baby's hips and legs should be flexed in a comfortable frog-like position). If it is long enough, the bottom corner can go over your baby's shoulder. Finally, take the last corner (right or left) and pull it toward you to make it tense. Then pull it across the baby's body, over the other arm, and tuck it in snugly underneath. Now, you literally have a little burrito bundle of joy! Make sure the blanket is not covering any part of her nose or mouth, as this can interfere with breathing.

Newborns feel comfortable and safe in a swaddle because it reminds them of when they were in the womb. A tight swaddle is also good for maintaining warmth. Your baby will let you know when she no longer wants to be swaddled by wriggling out of her swaddle or putting up more of a fight. This happens at different ages, but, in general, babies start to become more mobile between 3 and 6 months of age, when they discover how to roll. Once they are able to roll over, they should no longer be swaddled. A good alternative when swaddling just won't do anymore is to use a sleep sack or a wearable blanket sleeper. This looks like a small sleeping bag, with holes for the head and arms. Babies like it because it gives them some freedom in the crib when you put them down for a nap or for sleeping at night. It's also a great way to keep them warm, with a wearable blanket they can't get tangled up in! These are also advantageous because you avoid the use of a loose blanket in the crib, which may get caught when the baby rolls around or obstruct her airway if it's near her nose and mouth (for more information on safe sleeping, see chapter 14).

10. Is a pacifier okay?

Ah, the great pacifier debate. Here are the pros and cons.

Pros

☐ **Decreased risk of sudden infant death syndrome (SIDS)**
Why? We don't know for sure, but some experts believe that the sucking stimulates the breathing center in the brain, while others think that the

pacifier itself helps keep the airway open. In either case, the evidence is strong enough that the AAP now suggests that it is protective for a pacifier to be used when placing an infant to sleep during the first year after birth, but it should not be reinserted once the infant is asleep. If you're nursing, you can wait until breastfeeding is well-established before introducing a pacifier, usually around 2 weeks of age.

☐ **Babies soothe themselves by sucking**
Your breast is not meant to be a pacifier! If you have a baby with a strong urge to suck or a fussy baby who has been fed, burped, and changed, why not try the pacifier and see if it calms him down? My second son was a true pacifier baby. It kept him happy and calm, and that was reason enough for me!

Cons

☐ **Early use may interfere with breastfeeding**
It is sometimes difficult to identify and understand your baby's cues with a pacifier in his mouth, not to mention the fact that it is also easier to overlook his hunger cues. Additionally, some experts believe that infants may get confused since sucking on a pacifier (or even a bottle) involves a slightly different action than that required for breastfeeding—although most babies can learn to go back and forth easily.

□ **Overuse**

Infants quickly get used to the pacifier to soothe themselves and aid in sleep—a habit that is often hard to break down the road. Older infants who use pacifiers are more prone to getting colds, because they are accustomed to constantly sucking on and mouthing objects (the usual entry point for germs). In addition, pacifier use for longer than a year or two can interfere with tooth alignment and bite (just ask your pediatric dentist, whom your baby should start seeing once their first tooth arrives).

□ **Increased risk of ear infections**

There appears to be an association between pacifier use and an increased number of ear infections. Some experts feel that the constant sucking on the pacifier can push extra fluid into the middle ear, increasing a baby's chance of developing an ear infection.

So, what do you do? If you have a fussy baby or a baby who has a strong urge to suck, or if you want your baby to use a pacifier for falling asleep, wait until breastfeeding is well-established and your baby is gaining weight—usually around 2 to 4 weeks. Between 4 and 6 months, your baby needs to develop his own self-soothing skills for daytime and nighttime. (He should be sleeping through the night now; if not, see chapter 14, Sleep.) Therefore, the best time to get rid of the pacifier in my opinion is by 6 to 12 months of age. It's much easier to wean your baby off the pacifier at this age rather than waiting until your older infant or toddler has declared it his security object and won't go to sleep without it. You can also swap the pacifier for a blanky around 6 months of age. My third son was still addicted to his blanky for sleep at 22 months, but it won't affect his teeth, and he was happy and slept great, so it was a win-win. If you have an infant who doesn't like the pacifier, don't force it.

Body Parts

Babies come with lots of parts. From head to toe, there is a lot to cover but no instruction manual. Because this book is only meant to take on the most common questions, the list of parts covered may seem a bit random. Do you have other questions? Simply keep your own list and ask your pediatrician at your next well-baby visit. Should you find yourself with a more pressing question, pick up the phone and call your pediatrician.

11. I know my baby's belly button will be cute someday, but right now, it's just an alien-looking stump, with a little yucky fluid around it. When will the cord fall off?

Don't worry, that umbilical cord stump won't be around forever. The stump will typically fall off around

1 to 3 weeks after birth. In the meantime, make sure to keep the area clean and dry. It's also okay to just leave it alone—one less thing for you to do. If the area gets dirty from poop or pee, go ahead and clean it with a baby wipe or a little rubbing alcohol on a cotton swab. Many caregivers also prefer to fold the diaper down in front (or buy newborn diapers specially designed with the belly button area cut out) so the cord doesn't get irritated or rubbed the wrong way.

As the cord is falling off, it *is* normal to see some blood-tinged fluid or even dried blood a few days before and after the stump falls off. You may also notice a small, gooey lump (umbilical granuloma) at the base of the belly button. Other times, it can just be remnants of what we call Wharton jelly, a totally normal substance within the umbilical cord. But, either way, if you see or smell something funny, check with your pediatrician.

Two at-home treatments that many pediatricians recommend (always ask your own) to help it dry up and heal are:

1. Clean the granuloma with rubbing alcohol a few times a day for a few days.
2. Apply a pinch of table salt to the granuloma, cover with gauze, wash off after about 20 minutes, and dry the area. Try this twice a day for a few days.

Or your pediatrician may prefer to apply silver nitrate in the office. No matter which option you choose, the granuloma should eventually go away and look like a normal belly button soon. Sponge bathe your baby as needed until a day or two after the cord has fallen off and the belly button is dry and healed. Then you can start giving baths in a baby tub, rubber ducky and all—fun!

 Call your doctor if there is any redness on the skin surrounding the umbilical stump or if fluid or blood keeps leaking several days after the cord falls off. An infection at the site of the umbilical cord, although rare, can be very serious.

Nails ... To Cut or Not to Cut?

I don't know what's worse—looking at the self-inflicted scratches babies often get from their nails or trying to cut those nails! An easier (and sometimes safer) option is to file your baby's nails with a clean old-fashioned nail file or a motorized infant nail file. If you choose to cut or clip them and accidentally cut the skin (and we've all done it), apply pressure to stop any bleeding (which is usually minimal) and clean the wound well. Don't worry—your baby won't remember, and you can continue manicuring as needed. Although rarely an issue, call your pediatrician if the area won't stop bleeding or shows signs of infection, such as redness, swelling, or oozing. If possible, don't put gloves on the baby's hands. He needs to touch things to feel and learn about his environment.

12. My baby is congested. How can I help her breathe more comfortably?

Newborns and infants breathe mainly through their noses. Because their nasal passages are so tiny, a small amount of mucus can make a very loud noise. Even though your baby may sound really congested, don't let the noise bother you unless it interferes with your baby's eating or sleeping. If the nasal congestion does interfere with your baby's ability to eat or sleep, touch base with your pediatrician. Feeding your baby in an upright position may help. In addition, try the following techniques to relieve the congestion:

☐ Run a cool-mist humidifier in the room during sleep to keep the skin inside of the nose moist. Don't forget to clean the humidifier frequently so that germs are not collecting inside and spreading through the air!

☐ Remove visible mucus by placing a drop of nasal saline or breast milk in each nostril. Your baby may cough as the saline or breast milk drips from her nose, down the back of her throat—that's quite all right. Then gently suction out the mucus with a bulb syringe or nasal aspirator. Some nasal aspirators are battery operated, and others let you put one end of the tube in the baby's nostril and use your own mouth suction to draw out the mucus (don't worry, there's a filter, so no mucus actually gets in your mouth). If you can manage it or have an extra set of hands to help, hold one of your baby's nostrils closed while you suction the other nostril. Try suctioning when your baby is in a slightly upright position, as gravity can help the mucus drain. It's best not to suction more than a few times a day because it can irritate the inside of your baby's nose and worsen the congestion.

☐ Alternatively, after placing the saline in the baby's nose, give her some tummy time. As she moves her head up and down (and even if she cries), the mucus will be more likely to drain out on its own.

☐ Nasal saline drops can be bought or made (1/4 teaspoon of salt in 8 ounces of distilled water, sterile water, or boiled water that has been cooled down), and breast milk can be squirted or dripped right in.

☐ While nasal congestion usually is responsible for making a baby's breathing noisy, it is important to recognize signs of true troubled breathing that should be evaluated. A newborn normally breathes 30 to 60 times a minute (one breath every 1 to 2 seconds), which is much faster than an older child or adult breathes. If you feel that your baby is taking more than one breath per second, take a closer look.

☐ Can you see her tummy or the space between her ribs moving in and out with each breath (called retractions)?

☐ Do you hear wheezing (a high-pitched whistle) or other extra noises such as grunting with each breath?

☐ Is your baby's head bobbing as she breathes?

☐ Is she coughing?

☐ Is her nose flaring (nostrils widening) with each breath?

☐ Does her skin look blue?

 If the answer to any of these questions is "yes" or you simply can't tell the difference, call your pediatrician right away.

Baby Hiccups

Baby hiccups rarely bother your baby, but they often make parents really uncomfortable. The truth is that most babies hiccup from time to time. Often, getting a good burp and holding the baby upright after a feeding can decrease the chances of having hiccups. Also, feeding the baby while he is calm and not super hungry and agitated can help prevent hiccups.

If hiccups occur during a feeding, stop the feeding, burp the baby, and change the feeding position. Often, hiccups will disappear on their own in 5 to 10 minutes (they rarely last longer). If the hiccups don't go away on their own, try feeding again for a few minutes.

---

13. How can I prevent my baby from getting a flat head and needing a helmet?

To prevent your baby from developing a flat head (also known as *plagiocephaly*), while ensuring that your baby is sleeping in a safe environment on her back (for more on safe sleep, see chapter 14), alternate the side to which your baby's head is turned when she is sleeping. This helps keep any one part of your baby's relatively soft skull bones from flattening under pressure. You can also change the direction in which she is lying in her bassinet or crib, as well as alternate the side of your body that you feed and carry her on. This will help her get used to looking and turning her head in both directions.

In addition, remember that car seats are made for cars and are not intended to be used to carry a baby around in all day. The more time your little one spends in a car seat, bouncy chair, swing, or other device, with his head pressed back against a flat surface, the more likely his head will flatten.

Most importantly, when your baby is awake, remember to give him plenty of supervised tummy time—an activity that will serve to strengthen his head, neck, and upper body. You can begin tummy time in the first week after birth! Aim for 2 to 3 times a day, starting for just a few minutes and slowly increasing the amount of time as your baby gets used to and learns to enjoy it. Get down at the same level to encourage your baby to push up and lift the head and shake a toy to help guide him.

If you do notice that your baby's head seems flat in any way, show your pediatrician, who may recommend some specific positioning tips or exercises or, in extreme cases, if nothing is helping, refer you for an evaluation for a helmet to help reshape the head.

14. Should I circumcise my baby? How do I take care of his penis after the procedure?

Circumcision is an entirely personal decision, often influenced by religious or ethnic beliefs. Deciding whether to circumcise is completely your call. While there are some known medical benefits to the procedure, including a decreased risk of developing urinary tract infections, sexually transmitted infections, or penile cancer, as well as a reduced risk that a sexual partner will acquire cervical cancer later in your son's life, it's worth keeping in mind that some of these conditions can often be prevented in other ways. Ultimately, the decision might be made because of something one of my mentors always said: "Johnny should look like his daddy!"

Circumcision has been around for thousands of years, and although the technique and aftercare instructions may vary, most circumcisions ultimately turn out looking essentially the same. How you care for the penis after the procedure depends on how the circumcision is performed and the preference of the specialist provider performing it.

Circumcisions generally fall into 1 of 2 types, both of which should be performed by using some type of local anesthetic, so the newborn will not feel pain. The first uses the Plastibell, which is a ring that will fall off about a week after the circumcision. The second, and nowadays more common method, uses a non–ring-type metal clamp called a *Gomco, Sheldon,* or *Mogen clamp*. After the procedure, a thin piece of gauze may be left covering the incision site. If your provider advises using gauze, follow their directions. There will be some yellowish crusting or scabbing for about 7 to 10 days—don't worry, the skin will eventually heal and look normal. Until it has healed, your physician may recommend that you continue to cover the end of your baby's penis with petroleum jelly or another application of ointment at each diaper change and after a sponge bath to prevent the area from sticking to the diaper. If it does stick, don't freak out, just run a little warm water over the area so it unsticks.

 Call your pediatrician (or whomever performed your baby's circumcision) if your baby doesn't have a straight urine stream, if your baby hasn't peed for 8 hours after the circumcision (he may finally pee while you are dialing the phone), or if there is a lot of bleeding, pus, redness, or bruising.

15. How do I clean the foreskin if I don't circumcise my son?

Don't touch it! At least not yet, anyway. Retracting and cleaning a baby's foreskin can actually cause small tears in the tissue, which can lead to adhesions and possible problems later in life. Instead, simply wash the outside of your baby's foreskin with water (with or without a mild soap) as you would any other part of his body. As boys get older (usually around age 2), they begin having nighttime erections; as a result, the foreskin will gently stretch on its own. Any adhesions that may have formed will separate. That said, plenty of normal little boys are unable to retract the foreskin until at least the age of 4 or 5, at which time you can teach your son how to gently clean the foreskin and the head of the penis underneath it when he bathes. In due time, the foreskin will become easily retractable, and your son will be old enough to care for it on his own.

If there is ever any redness, swelling, or pain around your son's penis, bring it to the immediate attention of your pediatrician.

16. I found a red streak in my newborn's diaper. Could it be blood?

While it's certainly possible for a red streak in the diaper to be blood, it's usually not the most likely cause of such red discoloration.

☐ If the spot looks powdery, almost like blush or bronzer makeup, it may be urate crystals (little particles in urine that are seen when babies drink less the first few days after birth, often because mom's milk supply isn't fully in). Usually you can see the spots of these crystals right in the middle, with baby's urine surrounding it. Their appearance in the diaper is fairly common in the first few days after birth and nothing to worry about.

☐ If you have a boy who was circumcised, there may be a dark yellow or bloody stain on the diaper from the site of circumcision. Examine the tip of the penis for signs of infection and bleeding—call your pediatrician if you see something suspicious (see question 14, on page 27).

☐ If you have a girl, it is possible that the red stain is actually blood, but not the kind that warrants concern. Baby girls can have withdrawal bleeding in the first week after birth, similar to a woman's period. This occurs after birth because they are no longer exposed to mom's high estrogen levels. Again, it is nothing to worry about and will go away on its own.

 If you notice a red streak in your baby's diaper after the first week or have concerns at any time, you should see your baby's pediatrician. Try to bring a diaper with the stain or a close-up photo of it so your pediatrician can take a look.

CHAPTER 2

Breastfeeding

Many moms decide during pregnancy that they will nurse. Others are unsure and are looking for more information. And some new mothers don't make the decision to breastfeed until they first hold their new little one against their chest, skin to skin, and that perfect baby with an adorable tiny mouth grasps their nipple and begins to suckle. Whenever you decide, feel good in knowing that you are making an amazing difference in your baby's life, as well as your own.

Breastfeeding Basics

17. I want to breastfeed, but I'm worried I won't be able to do it. Where can I get help?

Although breastfeeding is natural, most babies aren't born experts (and neither are moms!). If you haven't seen somebody breastfeed in person, watching a few videos of a baby breastfeeding (even on YouTube) can help you get comfortable. Also, take advantage of

prenatal, labor and delivery, and breastfeeding classes
before you deliver so you understand the anatomy and
physiology of how your body actually makes the amazing breast milk that you will be feeding your little one.

It may take days (or even weeks) for you and your
little one to catch on, especially if your milk supply
is a little slow to come in. Try not to get discouraged.
Breastfeeding can take patience and hard work initially, but keep at it, because it's worth it for your baby's
health, as well as your own. Don't be afraid to ask for
help from day 1, if not before. Actually, it is common for
many new moms and even some experienced ones to
need some help breastfeeding. The American Academy
of Pediatrics (AAP) parenting book *New Mother's Guide
to Breastfeeding,* 3rd edition, is an easy, enjoyable read to
help guide new moms through nursing. You can talk to
your pediatrician about the ins and outs of breastfeeding even before you deliver, and you can ask for a list
of recommended resources in your community. Many
hospitals have lactation consultants available, and many
postpartum and nursery nurses are also trained to help.
Depending on where you live, there may also be local
lactation consultants, newborn care specialists, and postpartum doulas available in your community. Seek out an
Internationally Board Certified Lactation Consultant or
contact your local La Leche League chapter. Even one
meeting with a lactation specialist in the first few days
after having your baby can really pay off in the long run.
Additionally, many parenting support groups, breastfeeding centers, and stores have specialists available to
provide resources and help with nursing.

Breast Milk Is Truly Best

While breastfeeding can admittedly seem demanding because of the significant time commitment required (believe me, I know!), the benefits are well-documented and still growing, and the experience is priceless. Mother's milk provides immunity against bacteria and viruses (which means less sick time for your little one), is easiest for your baby to digest, is less expensive, and requires no preparation time (just pull up your shirt and feed). Additionally, it is uncommon for babies to be allergic to mother's milk. Studies show that breastfed babies have a lower rate of sudden infant death syndrome (SIDS), ear infections, respiratory infections, and diarrheal infections.

If you need one more reason to choose to breastfeed, especially during the first 100 days, breast milk's other role is to provide human milk oligosaccharides (aka HMOs or prebiotics) that feed good gut bacteria. In baby's intestines, these good bacteria—*Bifidobacterium infantis*—digest HMOs, releasing important nutrients that baby wouldn't get otherwise. The critical nutrients from HMOs help program baby's immune system and lower the risk of many childhood diseases such as food allergy, eczema, asthma, and diabetes.

And breastfeeding is not just good for baby; it has many documented benefits for mom, including a decreased risk of developing cancer and diabetes, as well as a faster return to prepregnancy weight. Breastfeeding uses up 300 to 500 calories per day—the equivalent of a 3-mile run! After all you've gone through, you deserve this nice payback!

18. My baby was born early. Can I still breastfeed?

Breast milk is still the optimal nutrition, even for pre-term (premature) babies. Breast milk composition changes, depending on when a baby is born and a baby's needs, so breast milk from a mom who delivers early contains a higher protein and nutrient composition than breast milk from a mom who delivers a full-term baby. However, if your baby was born very early, she may need extra vitamins, minerals, and calories added to your milk (eg, human milk fortifier) to help with her growth, as recommended by your neonatologist or pediatrician. Many neonatal intensive care units (NICUs) are even using donor breast milk banks to provide breast milk for a baby when a mom's milk isn't available.

Early initiation of breastfeeding, if okayed by your doctor, is best for establishing your milk supply. If your baby is not mature enough to breastfeed at first, you may be able to pump and supply milk to your baby until she is ready. Typically, babies born between 34 and 37 weeks of gestation are able to breastfeed, but they may need a little more practice to establish breastfeeding than babies born after 37 weeks. These babies can be sleepier or less coordinated than their full-term counterparts, making it harder for them to empty the breast. Ask for a lactation consult in the first day or two after birth to help evaluate the progress of you and your little one. Plenty of skin-to-skin contact (kangaroo care) and earlier initiation of pumping and hand expression, if milk production is an issue, can be helpful in increasing your supply.

Also, if your baby is in the NICU, talk to the nursing staff so you know the best time to hold, feed, and bond with your baby. Take advantage of all opportunities, such as when they change the isolette, to be with your little one. If your baby in the NICU requires special tube feeds, your pumped breast milk can still be used to provide your baby with all of the benefits of breast milk.

19. When does my "real" milk come in?

The first 2 to 3 days after your baby is born, you will produce yellowish, translucent fluid called *colostrum*. It is considered "liquid gold," is high in nutrients, and contains easy-to-digest proteins, fats, vitamins, minerals, and antibodies to protect your baby from disease. It also contains a mild laxative to help your baby stool and get rid of bilirubin, the stuff that causes jaundice (see question 101, on page 170). Colostrum is the perfect first food for your little one and just a few drops are all that she needs because her tummy is tiny (size of a large grape on day 1). Frequent feedings in the first few days, hand expressing milk prior to feeds, and rest (it's hard to find time, but you must), hydration, and proper nutrition will help increase your milk production. After about 3 days of breastfeeding, you will begin to produce transitional milk. Your breasts may begin to feel fuller and more tender. Continue to feed regularly, and by around 3 to 5 days, you should see a little white milk dripping from the corners of your baby's mouth or your nipple. You may even see it dripping from the opposite breast while you are feeding. Congratulations—your milk has come in! If you don't notice your breasts filling up with milk a week after your baby is born, call your doctor. Signs of good milk transfer to your baby include seeing your baby's chin drop with every suck, hearing swallowing noises, and having your baby produce wet and dirty diapers every day. Above all, the best sign that your baby is getting enough milk is weight gain. This will be measured at your pediatrician's office at every visit.

Breastfeeding—The Official Word

The AAP strongly supports breastfeeding as the optimal source of nutrition through the first year of your baby's life. The AAP recommends exclusively breastfeeding for around the first 6 months and then gradually adding solid foods while continuing to breastfeed, at least until your baby's first birthday. Breastfeeding can be continued for as long as you and your baby desire.

 Call your pediatrician if your baby isn't having at least 3 to 5 wet diapers and 3 to 4 dirty diapers (sometimes one diaper may have both urine and stool combined) per day by 3 to 5 days of age or if your baby looks more jaundiced (yellow tinge color to skin or eyes). This may be a sign that your baby isn't getting enough colostrum or breast milk.

20. Is feeding on a schedule or on demand better for newborns?

Initially, babies should feed approximately 8 to 12 times in 24 hours, which is roughly every 2 to 3 hours. However, sometimes your baby may want to feed more frequently, especially if she is cluster feeding. Breastfeed on demand as soon as your baby shows hunger cues, such as rooting (turning her head and opening her mouth in search of your breast), smacking her lips, making suckling motions, or bringing her hand to her mouth. Crying is a late sign of hunger, and it's best not to wait until your baby cries to feed. At this stage, babies may be harder to console and latching may be more challenging.

In the beginning, your baby may nurse on each side for 20 to 30 minutes, but after your milk comes in and she is gaining weight, she will get more efficient and take anywhere from 5 to 15 minutes per side. In general, the more often you breastfeed, the more milk you will produce, because your body will make what it thinks your baby needs. This can be demonstrated most impressively in breastfeeding mothers of twins, who will produce enough milk for both babies to feed and thrive! While some babies wake up every few hours on their own to feed, others may need a little coaxing. In the first few weeks, it's best to go with the flow and feed your baby as often as she wants, as this is the best way to establish a proper milk supply and ensure that your baby gets enough nutrition. Once your baby has gained weight, is over her birth weight, and is growing and developing well (usually around the 2-week checkup), you can let her sleep as long as she wants at night (turn off your alarm!).

If at this point you want to try more scheduled feedings (such as every 3 hours), go ahead and see how your newborn responds. Just know that some babies like to cluster feed during the day, eating as often as every hour or more frequently, but stretch out their nighttime feedings (which means more sleep for you!).

 If you are concerned about your newborn's feeding schedule or aren't sure if she is getting enough breast milk, see your pediatrician for a weight check between your normal well-baby examinations or whenever you feel it is needed.

Infant Vitamins

The AAP recommends that all breastfed infants be given vitamin D (400 IU or 10 mcg) once daily (available as infant vitamin drops), starting within the first few days after birth. This is because breast milk does not contain enough vitamin D (unless mom is taking 6,400 IU or 160 mcg of vitamin D daily), and a mom's vitamin D does not pass into breast milk well. Formula-fed babies also often need vitamin D supplementation, depending on which formula they drink and how much they are drinking. Ask your pediatrician if you have questions.

Vitamin D

It's important to note that vitamin D is fat soluble, so your baby can overdose if you accidentally give too much. If you aren't sure how much your baby consumed, or if you have questions, talk to your pediatrician, who will probably recommend waiting a few days or a week before restarting the vitamin.

Iron

Iron supplementation is also recommended for preterm (premature) babies, for infants starting iron rich solids later than age 4 months, or if an infant has a low hemoglobin level when tested around 12 months of age. Iron can be an important supplement if needed to help your baby make hemoglobin, which carries red blood cells throughout the body. Iron also supports brain development. Too much iron can also be harmful though, so always ask your pediatrician before starting your baby on an iron supplement.

Probiotics

Some pediatricians recommend feeding baby a daily infant-appropriate strain of probiotics to support the developing newborn gut, especially if the baby was born via C-section or mom or baby received antibiotics during or after labor. Contrary to popular belief, breast milk does not contain probiotics. Breast milk does contain prebiotics (HMOs) that feed specific good *Bifidobacterium* in your baby's intestines. Recent research shows that if such infant-specific good gut bacteria aren't present, the HMOs are not broken down into usable nutrients, and the HMOs are lost in the stool. If you have the right gut bacteria, they can provide your baby with long-term benefits. Not all probiotics are created equal, so make sure you always talk to your own pediatrician before giving your baby any supplement.

Pumping Pointers

21. Should I pump breast milk and offer it to my baby in a bottle? When do I start?

If you plan to return to work, or if you ever want to go out to dinner and a movie without your baby in tow, then yes! Pumping and storing breast milk to be served in a bottle at a later time can also give others the opportunity to feed and bond with your baby (and can give you a much-needed break).

Once you have established a good breastfeeding routine and feel comfortable enough to add something else to your to-do list (often when your baby is about 2 to 3 weeks of age or earlier if you are going back to work or if your pediatrician or lactation consultant recommends for low supply), you can begin to pump, store your breast milk, and introduce the bottle. The best time to pump and collect milk is often after the first morning feeding, since that is when you will often have extra milk because of nighttime hormones. Pump for 10 minutes on each side right after feeding.

If you wait too long to introduce the bottle, you run the risk that your baby may not take a bottle, and you'll get a panicked phone call from your sitter or child care provider to come right away. If he initially refuses the bottle because he prefers your breast, keep trying. It's often a good idea to have someone other than you give your baby a bottle at least once every few days (even while you are at home), so he remains familiar with it.

Breast pumps are manual or electric, but if you plan to pump frequently, an electric pump is the way to go. Medical insurance should cover an electric pump, so ask your obstetrician for a prescription and call your insurance company about a month before delivery and ask how to order. If you or your doctor feel you need something stronger, hospital grade pumps are often available for rent. Sound strange? Not really, once you discover that what you're really renting is the breast pump motor. All of the parts that touch you and your breast milk can be purchased brand new and sterile.

22. How do I store expressed breast milk?

Depending on the pump you have, breast milk can be pumped directly into special breast milk freezer bags or into bottles designed for refrigerator or freezer storage. To thaw breast milk for serving, hold the bag or bottle containing the frozen milk under warm running water or use a bottle warmer, but do not microwave it! Microwaving destroys the healthy infection-fighting antibodies in your milk, and it heats the milk unevenly, which could seriously burn a baby's mouth. To test the temperature of the milk, squirt a few drops on your own skin (your inner wrist is often recommended because the skin there tends to be thin and sensitive, like baby's skin). If you know how much milk your baby is likely to drink the next day, take that amount of frozen breast milk from the freezer the night before and place it in the refrigerator to thaw.

Be aware that you shouldn't refreeze thawed breast milk, so try to plan accordingly and only defrost what you think your baby will need.

So for how long is expressed breast milk good? Although you may remember "the rule of 4's" from previous guidance, here are the latest recommendations from the Centers for Disease Control and Prevention:

	Room Temperature 77°F (25°C) or colder	Refrigerator 40°F (4°C)	Freezer 0°F (-18°C) or colder
Freshly expressed/ pumped breast milk	Up to 4 hours	Up to 4 days	Up to 6 months is best Up to 12 months is acceptable
Thawed, previously frozen breast milk	1–2 hours	Up to 24 hours (1 day)	Never refreeze breast milk after it has been thawed
Leftover from a feeding (baby did not finish bottle)	Use within 2 hours after baby is finished feeding	—	—

Dr. Tanya's Tip

Create a Nursing Station

Choose a comfortable area in your home, such as a glider, rocking chair, couch, or armchair, and keep everything you need for a comfortable nursing session within arm's reach: a nursing pillow or support pillows, a glass of water (make sure to drink fluids every time you nurse), a snack (a whole-grain carbohydrate plus protein works well), your cell phone, your remote control, and anything else you'd like to have to ensure an uninterrupted nursing session.

Dr. Tanya's Tip
Pumping in the Workplace

☐ Talk to your supervisor, the Human Resources department, or other moms to find out what supplies, spaces, and break times are available for you so you can plan ahead. For example, is there a clean refrigerator for you to store pumped breast milk, or do you want to bring your own cooler? Is there an electrical outlet easily accessible, or do you need a battery pack?

☐ Looking at a photo of your baby or watching a video of her while you are pumping can help stimulate your letdown and increase the amount of milk you pump.

☐ The good news is that the "Break Time for Nursing Mothers" law is a federal law that requires employers to provide a reasonable amount of time for nursing mothers to express breast milk at work. Workplaces must also provide a private space for pumping that is not a bathroom. These provisions are protected up until 1 year after birth.

☐ It's always a good idea though to ask about your own company's policy and setup ahead of time to help you make a smooth transition when you return to work.

Common Concerns

23. My baby falls asleep at my breast. What can I do to help him stay awake while eating?

Falling asleep while eating is common, especially in the first few weeks. Nursing is very soothing to infants. That, combined with the warmth your baby feels snuggled against your chest, is an ideal combination to put anyone to sleep. In addition, some babies will tend to fall asleep in the first few weeks after birth when the flow of milk is slow—not necessarily because they have had enough to eat. If this is the case, gentle breast compression (use your opposite hand to hold your breast with the thumb on top and other fingers below) may help your baby get more milk and continue to nurse when he gets sleepy and his sucking slows down. It is important that your baby stay awake long enough to eat enough calories to gain weight and grow. Ideally, he will finish a full feeding, but during those first few weeks, this may be next to impossible each and every time you nurse him. Try stripping your baby down to only his diaper for nursing. Stroke his head, neck, or back or tickle his feet as needed to keep him awake. A good time to burp him or change his diaper is when you're shifting him between breasts; better yet, have Daddy or partner change it—a sure way to wake them both up.

 Call your pediatrician if your baby is so sleepy that you can't wake him to eat or if he has skipped 2 meals in a row.

Dr. Tanya's Tip

To Increase Milk Supply

☐ Stay hydrated (keep a water bottle within reach while nursing).

☐ Eat a balanced diet (about 500 calories more than you ate before pregnancy).

☐ Breastfeed regularly and alternate sides.

☐ Pump it up (pump an extra morning feeding if you have time).

☐ Get enough sleep (or as much as possible).

☐ Take a staycation with your baby to relax and focus on skin to skin, nursing, and cuddles.

Although there is not enough medical evidence to support the use of fenugreek capsules, Mother's Milk tea, goat's rue, blessed thistle, barley, oatmeal, breast milk cookies, or other whole-grain snacks to increase your milk supply, many moms swear that they really do work, and I looked forward to my afternoon oatmeal cookie snack to boost my milk supply.

 Always ask your pediatrician before using any medications or herbal supplements to make sure they are safe and don't have unwanted side effects.

24. My nipples are so sore that I cry during feedings. Help!

Been there! Sore, cracked nipples, most often caused by improper latch and vigorous or prolonged sucking, can be extremely painful and are the reason why some moms quit nursing. Enlisting the advice of a lactation consultant at the first sign of trouble, if not before, to learn proper latch and positioning techniques, along with good nipple hygiene, can usually prevent or resolve this irritating issue altogether. If you are experiencing pain, here are some tips to help your nipples heal and prevent further soreness.

- ☐ Even if you think your baby is latching on well, chances are your positioning may be slightly off. See the Proper Positioning for Latch tip on page 48. If that doesn't help, call a lactation consultant as soon as possible!
- ☐ Apply a lanolin (don't use if you have a wool allergy) or another breast cream/ointment/butter/balm labeled as safe for you and baby. This will help allow your breast to stay moist and heal.
- ☐ Express a few drops of breast milk and rub it over your nipple.
- ☐ Over the breast cream you've applied, wear a cotton bra, a loose-fitting top, and nipple shells—or even go bare when possible.
- ☐ Apply a cool compress or gel pads after nursing and a warm compress before nursing.

- ☐ Change nursing pads frequently.
- ☐ Try shorter feedings, or feed on one side at a time and give the other side a chance to heal.
- ☐ Change positions with every feeding to avoid repeated friction on the painful area of the nipple.
- ☐ Continue breastfeeding!
- ☐ Getting a neck and shoulder massage from your partner may not help the pain, but it sure doesn't hurt.

Call your pediatrician or lactation consultant if these remedies do not help within 24 to 48 hours, if the pain is getting worse, if a burning pain is experienced later on in breastfeeding (could be a yeast infection), or if your baby spits up blood-tinged milk (which may come from your cracked nipples).

Call your obstetrician if you develop the following:

- ☐ Increasing, persistent, or severe breast pain
- ☐ Fever
- ☐ Aches
- ☐ General flu-like symptoms

If you have these symptoms, you may have a breast infection (called *mastitis*) that requires treatment with an antibiotic. Continue breastfeeding (unless directed otherwise by your doctor) since the infection will not transfer to baby and nursing may actually help you clear your infection faster.

25. My milk is in, but now my breasts are so swollen and firm, I can't get my baby to latch. What can I do?

Normal breast fullness occurs around day 3 to 5 and is caused by a rapid increase in milk volume, combined with increased blood and lymphatic flow to the breast. This can lead to engorgement if your baby is feeding often enough or not fully emptying the breast. The breasts may have a shiny appearance and feel tender and firm to the touch. The treatment is simply to feed more often to remove more milk. However, this can be a struggle when the breasts become so firm that your baby can't latch well. Tips to reduce engorgement include using warm compresses prior to feeds, massaging the breast gently, expressing milk by hand, or using a breast pump for a few minutes prior to a feeding. This can soften up the area around the nipple, allowing your baby to latch on and feed effectively. If she is still unable to nurse, the milk can be removed by hand expression or pumping and then given to her. Frequent feedings (every 2–3 hours) are the key to preventing future engorgement.

Proper Positioning for Latch

Improper latch can cause pain and blisters and really interfere with breastfeeding. Here is a walk-through on proper latching, straight from my own childbirth and lactation educator, Polly Gannon, CCE, CLE, ANCS.

Sit up straight and comfortably, with your back supported and a nursing stool under your feet to elevate them. Use regular pillows or a nursing pillow on your lap to help elevate the baby and provide support. Position your baby chest to chest so she is facing you, with her ear, shoulder, and hip in alignment. The goal is to put the baby on the breast—not put the breast in the baby's mouth. Hold your baby with one arm and your hand supporting the back of the neck (see the cross-cradle hold, as described in the answer to the next question). Her nose should be close to your nipple. Allow your baby's head to tilt back so she's looking at your nipple. Tease the baby's lips with your nipple. Wait for her to open her mouth widely (like a fish). When she does, bring her closer to you and put most of the areola (the darker part of the nipple) into her mouth. It's okay to gently pull down on her lower lip to get a symmetrical "fish lip" latch. Any of the positions described in the answer to the next question work well, but initially, the cross-cradle or football hold is often easiest.

When your nipple comes out of your baby's mouth, it should look round—not creased or dented, like used lipstick. If it is, that means your latch isn't perfect, and you're headed for a blister. A feeling of tugging is normal, especially for the first 15 to 30 seconds, but pain is a sign that you should ask for help.

If your baby latches on, but it's very uncomfortable for you, don't continue to suffer. Break the latch and try again. The best way to break a latch is to hook your pinky finger near the edge of the baby's mouth and gently pull to release the suction. If you pull your baby off the breast without breaking the suction, it can cause even more pain and damage to your nipple.

26. What's the best way to position my baby so we are both comfortable during a feeding?

In the beginning, you may become so focused on supporting your baby that you neglect your own comfort. It takes practice and patience to find a position that is comfortable for both you and your baby, but it's worth the effort! There is no one right way, but I'll review a few common holds here. To start, get in a comfortable seated or slightly reclined position. Have plenty of pillows handy to help support your baby and your arms. Having your feet resting on a raised surface can prevent you from leaning forward, hunching over, and straining your neck or back. In any position, think about bringing your baby to your breast, not the other way around. In any position, the baby's ear, shoulder, and hip should be in a straight line. Remember, the more comfortable and relaxed you are, the more enjoyable it will be for both of you.

☐ **Cradle:** This is a classic breastfeeding position, so called because you cradle your baby's head in the crook of your arm. To nurse on the left breast, for example, her head will be in the crook of your left arm. Hold her so that she is facing you with your left arm supporting her back. You may tuck her lower arm under yours. It may be hard to guide baby's mouth to your nipple in this position initially, but it should get easier once she has better head control. This position is a favorite with older babies and their moms.

☐ **Cross-cradle:** This position uses the opposite arm from the one in the cradle position. For example, to feed on your left breast, support your baby with your right arm, with your hand under her head and her body resting on your arm. This allows a little more control to guide her mouth to your breast and is a great position for many newborns.

☐ **Football:** Similar to the way you would hold a football, you tuck your baby under your arm on the same side you're feeding from. Rest your arm on a pillow and use your hand to support your baby's head and guide her to the breast. This position may work best for moms with larger breasts or moms who have had C-sections because you avoid placing any pressure on the stomach.

☐ **Side-lying:** Ideal for nursing in bed, you lie on your side and bring baby to your breast, cradling her head with either arm. You will want to have plenty of pillows to support your head and back. To find the right angle, you may need to lift the breast slightly to align it with your baby's mouth.

☐ **Laid back:** This is a more relaxed method, where you are leaning back on a well-supported surface and baby's whole body is lying on you. She can be in any position, as long as the entire front of her body is resting on you. Her cheek may first rest on your breast, and then you can guide her as needed to find the nipple. This position allows gravity to help keep your baby in position and can be less stressful for some mothers.

27. My baby spits up often. Is this normal?

All babies spit up once in a while, but some babies spit up more frequently, leading moms to wonder if their newborn is allergic to something in the adult diet that is passing through the breast milk. In many instances, spit-up is caused not by an allergy but by reflux or a baby's getting too much milk too quickly. Reflux is discussed in more detail in chapter 4 but, simply put, some of the milk that your baby drinks (along with stomach acid) manages to work its way back up from the stomach. If your baby seems to gulp and gasp, try taking her off the breast for a little rest or even a burp before putting her back on. Have a burp cloth handy to catch the milk that happens to spurt out. Giving smaller feedings more frequently, such as with one breast instead of both at each feeding, burping halfway through a feed, and keeping your baby in an upright position for 10 to 15 minutes after a feeding instead of laying her down can also help. Despite your best efforts, the fact of the matter is that spitting up is often a part of newborn life. If this is the case, keep stacks of burp cloths everywhere and don't forget an extra change of clothes for baby (as well as for you) when going out.

In some instances, your baby may develop an allergy to something that you are eating. The most common offenders are milk and soy products, but eggs, nuts, wheat, fish, shellfish, citrus, and others are also possibilities. Always talk to your physician before restricting your diet, as proper nutrition is essential for breastfeeding.

If your baby's spit-up seems excessive, is projectile (shoots across the room), is bright green, or contains blood, or if she seems very uncomfortable or has extreme crying or poor weight gain, call your pediatrician. In addition, if there is any diarrhea, blood in the stool, or vomiting, an allergy is more likely to be a culprit, so check with your pediatrician.

Excess Gas?

Certain foods that make you gassy may also cause gas in your baby and make him uncomfortable. A few culprits include spicy dishes, beans, and cruciferous veggies including broccoli and cauliflower. Usually symptoms lessen as your baby grows and you can then try reintroducing these foods into your diet.

28. I have a cold. Should I continue nursing?

Absolutely. Your breast milk can actually help protect your infant from catching your cold. Your body begins making antibodies as soon as you become infected. These protective antibodies are passed to your baby through your breast milk. Chances are that your baby was exposed to your illness before you even started feeling sick, so if you stop nursing, there is an even greater chance that she will catch your cold. It's still a good idea to wash your hands before touching your baby and try to avoid kissing her face or directly coughing or sneezing on her. Even before COVID, sick parents and caregivers were often advised to wear a mask to decrease the chance of spreading illness to baby.

 If your doctor recommends that you stop nursing because of a serious illness, medication, or treatment that you need, talk with your pediatrician. There may be a way to continue feeding your baby your breast milk.

29. Can I have a glass of wine or a cup of coffee or take over-the-counter medications while I'm breastfeeding?

What goes in, must come out! What you eat or drink will pass through to your breast milk in some amount and can potentially affect your baby.

You may be surprised to know that occasional, minimal alcohol consumption is actually okay. It can be dehydrating though, so drink extra water to keep up your milk supply. The best time to have that glass of wine is right after you finish nursing or pumping and at least 2 hours before your next feeding or pumping session. That way, your body has as much time as possible to get rid of the alcohol, and less will reach your baby.

Although you don't have to quit caffeine cold turkey, it's worth pointing out that while caffeine may perk you up, it may also cause fussiness and wakefulness in some babies. It is therefore best to limit your overall intake of caffeine, whether your preference is coffee, tea, caffeinated soda, or even chocolate. Although some experts say that up to 3 cups a day may be fine, it's probably best to stick with the minimum amount you need. It's also best to have coffee, soda, or chocolate earlier in the day so any caffeine that does pass through won't interfere with your baby's nighttime sleep.

When it comes to medications or herbal supplements, as always, you'll want to check with your baby's pediatrician before taking any. Also, make sure your own physician knows you are breastfeeding before any medication is prescribed for you. Luckily, most over-the-counter pain medications such as acetaminophen (Tylenol) and some cold medications (when taken in appropriate amounts) are safe while breastfeeding. It is important to note that any medication that dries up your secretions or nasal congestion (such as decongestants and antihistamines) may have the same effect on your breast milk, especially if taken regularly.

CHAPTER 3

Formula Feeding

For many, the decision to breastfeed or formula feed is based on comfort level, lifestyle, and specific medical situations. If you are unable to breastfeed or decide it's not for you, infant formula is a healthy alternative. You may even choose to supplement breastfeeding with formula. Formula will provide your baby with all the nutrients he needs to grow and thrive. Plenty of successful adults were formula fed as infants and keep up just fine with their breastfed counterparts. Talk to your doctor or lactation consultant if you're having trouble deciding between methods and want to learn more.

What may be even more difficult than deciding whether to use formula is which formula to use and how to feed it to your little one. You may be bombarded with choices. Many formulas contain docosahexaenoic acid (DHA) and arachidonic acid (ARA), most have iron, and others are organic or have probiotics. In this chapter, I will attempt to make sense of the smorgasbord of infant formulas available.

Formula Facts

30. There are so many different formulas to choose from. Where do I start?

Ever wish there were a simple mathematic formula that would allow you to calculate which infant formula is best for your baby? Unfortunately, it's not that easy. The good news is that any major-brand formula on the market should be fine, and most babies do very well on the first one they are given. Your pediatrician can also help you select an appropriate formula for your baby.

Here's the scoop on infant formula.

Main Types

☐ **Cow's milk based:** This is recommended as the formula of choice for infants not receiving breast milk. You will find this to be the most commonly marketed type of formula in stores. Some companies sell variations that are meant to help with reflux, gassiness, or other digestive problems, but they are generally not very different in composition because they have to meet important and strict standards set by the US Food and Drug Administration (FDA). Most infants grow and develop very well on standard cow's milk–based formula.

☐ **Soy based:** Soy protein is used instead of cow's milk protein and is naturally lactose free. Soy formula is a good alternative to milk-based formula for vegetarian families and for some infants who are allergic to or intolerant of cow's milk protein. However, many babies who are allergic to cow's milk are also allergic to soy protein, so we don't advise switching formulas for this reason without consulting your pediatrician. While no convincing evidence exists that soy-based formulas prevent the development of allergies, parents also don't need to worry that they are linked to early puberty or other issues.

☐ **Protein hydrolysate and elemental:** Often referred to as *hypoallergenic formulas,* these are made specifically for infants with a severe allergy to standard cow's milk and soy protein–containing formulas. The proteins in both these types of formulas are broken down into basic components that may make them less likely to cause food allergies. Unfortunately, although these formulas may be digested more easily, they are also generally more expensive. It's best to only use these formulas when medically necessary because of an allergy or a recommendation by your pediatrician, allergist, or gastrointestinal physician.

Additives

☐ **Iron:** Iron is vital for blood and brain development. Contrary to popular belief, the amount of iron in formula should not cause constipation. More importantly, low-iron formulas do not contain enough iron for a baby's growing needs (brain and body). Always buy iron-fortified formula! Babies who consume iron-fortified formulas usually do not need extra iron supplements.

☐ **DHA and ARA:** These are 2 fatty acids (lipids) that occur naturally in breast milk and are thought to be important in brain and eye development. They can also be found naturally in fish oils and eggs and are considered "good fats." DHA and ARA have now been added to most formulas.

☐ **Probiotics:** Similar to those found in yogurt with live bacteria cultures, probiotics, or "friendly bacteria," have been added to some infant formulas. The most common strains you might see on labels are *Bifidobacterium and Lactobacillus.* Some research has shown that probiotics may have a benefit in preventing and treating certain types of illness.

☐ **Organic:** They are certified to be free of pesticides, antibiotics, and growth hormones. Only time and research will tell if there is any medical benefit when it comes to a manufactured food product such as formula, but if buying organic is important to you, it is fine. Just make sure you buy a reputable brand to ensure that it contains everything your baby needs to grow and develop and has met the strict standards set forth by the FDA.

Preparations

☐ **Ready to feed:** As the name states, your baby can drink this formula as is. Once opened, it can be stored in the refrigerator for 48 hours. Although convenient for travel if you can't or don't want to carry water for mixing, the bottles are heavy to carry around and are often more expensive than powdered formula.

- ☐ **Liquid concentrate:** This type of formula is easy to mix—you simply add equal parts of the liquid formula and water, shake, and feed. Again, it is heavier to haul around in your baby bag and is a slightly more expensive option than powder.
- ☐ **Powder:** This preparation is the most commonly used and least expensive option. Also, powder is fairly light to carry. The mixing ratio for formula is 2 ounces of water for 1 scoop of powder formula. Simply shake or stir and then serve.

European/Australian Formula

European and Australian formulas and the new US companies manufacturing "European or Australian" formulas are becoming more popular. Some caregivers report choosing them because of the perception that the formulas are of higher quality, because European or Australian formula standards are different, or because they offer other options such as goat's milk or milk from pasture-raised cows, which are rare or nonexistent in a US Food and Drug Administration–regulated form in the United States. It's important to always talk to your pediatrician about formula choice to ensure that there are enough vitamins and nutrients for your growing baby. In addition, please read the package instructions carefully, as many European and Australian formulas have a different size scoop as well as different mixing instructions (usually 1 European scoop to 1 ounce of water).

31. If I premix my powder formula with water, how long will it last?

Most infant formulas can last up to 24 hours when refrigerated after mixing. Formula left out at room temperature should be used within 1 hour. It's a good idea to toss any unused formula after feeding and make a fresh bottle at the next feeding. See the following Dr. Tanya's Tip on a great way to travel with powder formula, without having to mix it ahead of time!

Dr. Tanya's Tip
Drinking on the Go

Premeasure scoops of powder formula into a dry bottle for storage in your baby bag. When it's time to feed your baby, just add the appropriate amount of bottled water (2 ounces of water per 1 scoop of powder formula), shake, and serve. Room-temperature water is fine. Some formulas now offer small on-the-go powder packets for convenience too!

32. What kind of bottles should I buy?

Bottles come in different shapes and sizes, are made of different materials, and a few even have disposable liners inside. Glass bottles are free of BPA (bisphenol A), a chemical used in some plastic storage containers that may leach into food and beverages over time. However, glass containers can crack and chip, so they need to be checked often. Almost all newer plastic bottles are "BPA-free" and labeled as such. Because some scientific studies show that infants can be vulnerable to the health effects of BPA exposure, only use bottles that are BPA free. There are also stainless-steel infant bottles on the market that are extremely strong but heavy, and it can be challenging to measure the amount of liquid that is in the bottle. As your little one grows, his appetite will gradually increase, so you will eventually need the bottle to hold more than just 4 ounces! Another thing to consider is that many bottles now have a built-in venting system that helps limit the amount of air the baby swallows to help prevent gassiness. Make sure to follow the instructions as the bottle position is important to allow the air to vent.

33. How do I choose a bottle nipple? How often should it be replaced?

Nipples often come in different numbers or "stages" to reflect the size of the nipple's hole, which affects the flow rate (ie, slow, medium, or fast) of formula or breast milk coming out. For example, fast flows may cause younger babies to gag or may simply give them more than they can handle, whereas slower flows may frustrate some babies and cause them to suck harder and gulp too much air. Different nipple shapes also may be advertised to fit the inside of your baby's mouth (orthodontic nipples), to resemble the natural shape of a mother's breast, or to be easier for preemies to use. You may need to try a few different varieties or brands before finding one that works best for your baby.

Start with the "stage 1" or "level 1" nipples, which are slower flow and typically perfect for a full-term newborn. Replace the nipple as your baby is ready to move on to the next size or when the nipple looks cracked, discolored, or thin. If an older infant is sucking on a nipple for long periods of time, but not getting enough volume, it may be time to increase the nipple size.

34. Should I boil the water I use to mix my baby's formula?

That depends on your local water supply. In most areas in the United States, regular tap water is fine, but in some areas—primarily those where well water is used—you may be advised to boil tap water for 1 minute to sterilize it before using it to make formula. You can also buy bottled water.

In addition, you should determine whether there is fluoride in your area's water supply and talk to your pediatrician or pediatric dentist about your baby's fluoride needs. Although some fluoride is important for developing teeth that have not yet made their appearance, too much fluoride can cause problems, especially for babies younger than 6 months.

35. Do I need to warm the formula before giving it to my baby?

Room-temperature formula is fine for babies and easier for you. Although it's not necessary, if you would like to warm the formula, go ahead. Use a bottle warmer, run the bottle under warm running water, or let it sit in a pot of warm water. Do not microwave it, as this can cause hot pockets in the formula that may inadvertently burn your baby. Always make sure to shake the bottle before testing the temperature (a few drops on your inner wrist works well), because some areas in the bottle may be warmer than others. As your baby gets older, transition to mixing your formula with room-temperature water. Remember that if your baby gets used to drinking warm formula, you will run into problems when you are out and don't have a way to warm the formula to the desired temperature. It's all about what your baby gets used to.

Formula for Toddlers?

Toddler formulas are now available from a variety of formula companies. Made for 9- to 24-month-olds, these formulas do have extra vitamins and nutrients compared with regular whole milk. But are they really necessary? Reports have shown that in most cases, they aren't. If your child is eating a balanced diet and growing and developing well, regular whole milk is sufficient for your child's needs after her first birthday. Plus, regular milk costs less than many of these toddler formulas. In specific cases, if your pediatrician is concerned about your toddler's growth or diet, then he or she may recommend that you give formula for a longer period.

Unexpected Upsets

36. My baby is fussy and gassy and spits up often. Should I switch formulas?

Some babies are fussy and gassy and spit up more often than others. It's rarely dangerous, but it isn't exactly fun, either. Try the following tips and tricks before you jump to switching formulas:

- ☐ Walk with your baby or sit in a rocking chair to try various positions.
- ☐ Try burping your baby more often during feedings.
- ☐ Place your baby belly down across your lap and rub his back.
- ☐ Hold your baby upright for 15 or 20 minutes after each feeding. Put your baby in a swing—the motion may have a soothing effect.
- ☐ Put your baby in an infant car seat in the back of the car and go for a ride. The vibration and movement of the car often calm a baby.
- ☐ Ask your pediatrician about trying an infant-specific probiotic, as fussiness and excess gas can be a sign of insufficient good gut bacteria (newborn gut deficiency).

While symptoms of spitting up, crying after feedings, and excessive gassiness do not indicate a true allergy, in some cases they suggest an intolerance to a specific type of formula. See the answer to the following question for more signs of how to tell the difference. Although some babies seem to show a preference for a specific type or brand of formula, most do fine on the first formula they are given. For parents who are constantly switching formulas on a quest for that one magic formula, when they eventually find it, often the reason is that their infant is older and has outgrown the symptoms.

37. How do I know if my baby is allergic to milk-based formula?

Signs of a true cow's milk protein allergy are usually not subtle. You may see hives (a blotchy, raised, and red skin rash), eczema, facial swelling, vomiting, or difficulty breathing. Another type of formula allergy may produce bloody diarrhea and cause poor weight gain. Some babies, however, may have more mild symptoms, such as spitting up, fussiness, and changes in stool pattern. Always talk to your pediatrician if you are concerned that your baby may have a milk or other food allergy.

 If your baby has any trouble breathing, facial swelling, vomiting, or hives, call your pediatrician immediately. The doctor may recommend that your baby be given a hypoallergenic formula.

Baby Bottle Tooth Decay

Please don't put your baby to bed with a bottle. No matter how you feed your baby (breast or bottle, once teeth start coming in, it is recommended to gently brush teeth after her last nighttime feed (see question 134 on how to brush). Falling asleep while drinking milk or juice can lead to cavities because the liquid pools around the teeth and provides a place for bacteria to grow. In addition to being bad for primary (baby) teeth, there can also be damage to future permanent teeth. Also, falling asleep while drinking increases your baby's chance of developing ear infections. Bottle propping (when a bottle is propped up to allow a child to drink without a parent holding it) is just as bad and may also lead to choking as the milk continues to flow out. Don't start an unnecessary feeding habit that often leads to a bad sleeping habit—both of which are difficult to break.

CHAPTER 4

Beyond Bottles and Breastfeeding

Starting Solid Foods

What kind of pediatrician and parent would I be if I didn't take this opportunity to stress the importance of proper nutrition? As a parent, you are your child's best role model when it comes to healthy eating. Kids like to eat what they see their parents eating. And if you get excited about a particular item, they will too. That's how I got my son to eat broccoli every night for dinner when he was a toddler. I'm not going to tell you that it's easy. After his first grilled cheese sandwich, he was hooked, and that was all he wanted. So—mysteriously—all of the bread and cheese in the house disappeared for a week, until he forgot about it! If the only choices available to your child are healthy ones, most older infants and toddlers will take to eating healthier options and learn to love them. I have toddlers in my practice who eat high-fiber cereal with raisins and milk and drink a cup of water for breakfast almost every day.

In the Beginning

38. Should I give my baby water?

There is no need to give newborns any water, sugar water, electrolyte solutions (such as Pedialyte, Enfalyte, or LiquiLytes), or juice, unless directed by your pediatrician. Doing so may interfere with your newborn's essential nutrition needs. Breast milk or formula is all your baby needs at this age.

Once your infant is ready for solid foods, which will be around 6 months of age, you can start introducing water at mealtimes. Getting your infant used to the taste of water (instead of sweet beverages) will help create a healthy habit for life. Gradually work up to giving 4 to 8 ounces of water a day in a cup (open, straw, or sippy), beginning around 6 months of age.

39. How can I be sure that my newborn is getting enough to eat?

In addition to following how much and how often your baby eats, it is helpful to track his weight, as well as how much he pees and poops. During the first 2 weeks after birth, breastfed babies feed 8 to 12 times a day, about 15 to 20 minutes on each breast. Formula-fed babies typically drink approximately 1 or 2 ounces every 3 to 4 hours (the amount at each feeding will increase after the first week or two). Your pediatrician will closely follow your baby's weight since newborns may lose up to 10% of their birth weight in the first week. By the end of the second week, however, they usually gain it back. After that, babies usually gain about an ounce a day, for the first few month. Most babies double their birth weight by 5 or 6 months of age and triple it by 1 year. If your baby is losing too much weight or not gaining weight appropriately, then your pediatrician may ask you to come in for more frequent visits to monitor your baby's growth more closely.

In the first week, a good way to determine if enough is going in is to keep track of what is coming out. For the next few weeks, your baby should have at least 5 wet diapers and 3 dirty diapers a day. Don't forget that many times a diaper has urine and stool mixed together.

Here is a chart to show you what kind of "diaper output" your newborn should have in his first days.

Day	Wet Diapers (Urine)	Dirty Diapers (Stool)
Day 1	1 or more	1 or more
Day 2	3 or more	2 or more
Day 3	4 or more	3 or more
Day 4	5 or more	3 or more

 Let your pediatrician know if your baby is having fewer wet and dirty diapers than what is listed in this chart or if your baby has a change in his usual pattern. A significant decrease in wet diapers may indicate illness or not enough fluid intake.

Baby Burps

Most babies need to burp for the first few months to help get rid of swallowed air. Some babies feel better having a burp halfway through a feeding, while others are fine waiting until the full feeding is over. And some babies do well burping before a feeding to get gas out and allow space for what they are about to drink. Of course, you won't always be able to get a burp out of him. If you've been trying to burp him for 5 minutes and he seems comfortable, it's okay to give up. Here are several burping techniques you can try.

1. Sit your baby on your lap and lean his weight slightly forward against one of your hands (making sure to support his chest and head) and gently pat his back. You can also gently rotate his body around in a circular fashion to help release some of the trapped gas.
2. Drape him over your shoulder and gently pat and rub his back.
3. Lay him tummy-side down over your lap. With your other hand, gently pat and rub his back.

Spit-up Happens!

For some babies it happens often. Most of the time, the spit-up looks just like the milk they drink, and it happens soon after feedings. Other times, it is curdled like old milk or smelly like vomit and can come up an hour or two after feedings. Spit-up is caused by taking too much volume in at once or by reflux (see question 40, on page 73).

It should not be forceful, although if you are holding your baby up on your shoulder, it may shoot over your shoulder and down your back (if you're lucky, it will miss your hair!). So buy burp cloths by the dozens and keep them everywhere.

Spitting up also shouldn't cause a great deal of discomfort for your baby. In fact, your baby may feel better after a good spit-up. As she gets older, the spitting up will improve and usually resolves by 6 to 12 months of age.

Call your doctor if the spit-up seems forceful (shoots across the room), your baby seems to be in pain, or you notice any blood or greenish color in the spit-up or any increase in frequency or intensity. Also call if her belly looks swollen or distended or feels hard. In addition, tell your pediatrician if you notice that your baby doesn't seem to be gaining weight or is having fewer wet and dirty diapers, as these may be signs that not enough of what she eats is staying down. If you think your baby's spit-up is not normal, it may be useful to keep a log and take photos if possible of spit-ups for a week to show your pediatrician. For example, take note of what the spit-up looks like, when it happens (time of day, during or after a feeding), and the estimated volume (the entire volume of the feeding, half the feeding, or just a few drops).

40. What is reflux? I see this word in a lot of parenting magazines.

Reflux is the name used for spit-up caused by the stomach contents going "the wrong way" out of the stomach. It is common in babies because a baby's feeding tube (esophagus) is short, and the muscles (sphincter) located at the bottom of the feeding tube/ top of the stomach are relaxed and floppy. This allows food in the stomach to come back up and out of the mouth. Hence the spit-up!

As long as your baby is a "happy spitter" and is feeding, growing, and developing well, usually no treatment is needed. The feeding tube will lengthen, and the sphincter muscles will naturally tighten as he grows, so the spitting up or reflux usually resolves by about 1 year of age. In the meantime, giving your baby smaller, more frequent feedings and holding him upright for 10 to 15 minutes after a feeding will help.

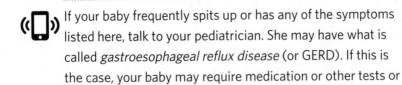 If your baby frequently spits up or has any of the symptoms listed here, talk to your pediatrician. She may have what is called *gastroesophageal reflux disease* (or GERD). If this is the case, your baby may require medication or other tests or treatment. Symptoms include the following:

- ☐ Your baby is not feeding well or is not gaining weight appropriately.
- ☐ Your baby develops respiratory symptoms such as coughing, choking, or wheezing during or after feeding.
- ☐ Your baby seems uncomfortable, cries, or arches her back after a feeding (she may not always spit up).
- ☐ The spit-up is projectile (it literally shoots across the room).
- ☐ The spit-up is green. (This may indicate a different problem that requires immediate attention, so call your pediatrician right away!)

In such cases, your pediatrician may recommend changing the consistency of your baby's formula or breast milk (using a thicker formula or adding a small amount of rice cereal or oatmeal) or even starting medication to help with the reflux. It's also important to note that reflux peaks between 2 and 3 months of age, so the volume of spit-up might worsen before it gets better.

Solids and Such

41. When can my baby start eating solid foods?

The American Academy of Pediatrics (AAP) and most pediatricians recommend starting solids around 4 to 6 months of age, when caregiver and baby are both ready.

So, how do you know when your baby is ready? All babies grow and develop at slightly different rates, and although some cultures start solids in the first few months with no apparent harmful effects, this isn't generally recommended because your infant isn't developmentally ready for solid food yet.

First, your baby needs to have good head control, which most infants demonstrate in the 4- to 6-month age range. In addition, she needs to be able to move the food with her tongue from the front to the back of her mouth, which is also something that occurs from 4 to 6 months of age. If you put a small amount of pureed food (such as pureed avocado, carrots, or peas) on her tongue and she pushes it out of her mouth (because of the tongue thrust reflex), she may not be developmentally ready for solid food. But if she is drinking more than 36 ounces a day, it's probably time for a bit of solid nutrition. Another sign you will begin to notice around this age is that she may pull away from the breast or bottle to look around for other interesting things to do (or eventually eat). She may also watch you intently as you eat and put her own hands near or in her mouth.

As long as your baby is at least 4 months old and meeting most of these criteria, go ahead and talk to your pediatrician about trying solid foods. If your baby was premature, it may take longer than 4 months for her to be ready, and that's okay. If she spits the food out, simply wait a few days or a few weeks and try again.

Remember to touch base with your pediatrician at the 4- or 6-month checkup to get advice about starting solid food.

Dr. Tanya's Tip
Toss the White Rice Cereal

Years ago, white rice cereal was the first food fed to babies. However, times have changed, and we now know there really isn't much nutritional benefit to feeding your baby any white cereal. If you do choose to feed your baby cereal (or mix it with a healthy veggie or nut butter), I prefer whole-grain choices, such as oatmeal, quinoa, and brown rice. Cereal is fortified with iron and zinc, so if your baby isn't eating chicken

or meat around 6 to 8 months of age, then it's a good idea
to add a whole-grain cereal to your infant's diet to ensure
she gets enough iron and zinc for growth and development.
As with all foods, if you start your infant out on whole-grain
cereal, bread, and pastas, then that's what he will eat when he
is older. Whole grains are higher in fiber and nutrients and are
therefore a much healthier lifelong dietary choice than white
grain alternatives.

42. How should I introduce solids to my baby, and what food should I start with?

There are no strict guidelines anymore regarding the
order in which solid foods should be introduced. The
goal is to offer your baby a wide variety of healthy,
whole foods in a form that she can handle (and not
choke on). Try mashed avocado, pureed vegetables or
fruits, pureed chicken, yogurt, pureed or scrambled
and fork-mashed eggs, whole-grain baby cereals, and
pureed fish—all good foods to feed your baby. You can
steam, bake, or boil foods and puree or mash them
with a fork by adding a little breast milk or water to
thin the consistency if needed. Start by giving your
baby a food with a soup-like consistency once a day.
Over time, you can gradually thicken the consistency
and increase your solid food offerings to 2 and, later,
3 times a day. You can also cut soft/steamed pieces
of food into long, thin slices that can fit in your
baby's palm.

If you prefer to buy baby foods, a wide variety of healthy options is available at the store or online (what could be easier than delivered to your door?). From foods with a long shelf life to small-batch organic, cold-pressed, or frozen options, just keep it all balanced and healthy, with no added sugar, preservatives, or unpronounceable ingredients.

When you're out and about, I find it easy to order a side of avocado or banana. These are easy to mash with a fork and feed to an infant. As your baby gets older, food can become lumpier in consistency, and by around 8 to 12 months of age, your baby will begin to be able to pick up small pieces of soft food to eat by himself. The goal is to gradually get your baby to eat regular, healthy foods, while sitting at the table with the rest of the family 3 times a day, by around 1 year of age.

43. How do I know if my baby is allergic to a specific food?

Food allergies are more common in children with a family history of food allergies or other allergic conditions, such as asthma, hay fever, or eczema. As you introduce new foods into your baby's diet, watch out for any signs of a potential food allergy, and let your pediatrician know if you see any symptoms.

Food allergy symptoms can be mild, such as a dry, scaly rash (eczema) and a blotchy rash (hives). More severe signs include full-body hives, facial swelling, trouble breathing, vomiting, diarrhea, and anaphylaxis (a life-threatening reaction).

Call your doctor right away if you notice any of these severe symptoms. If your infant is having trouble breathing, call 911.

With food allergies on the rise, there is now research and guidance on food allergy prevention for your baby or for siblings of a child with food allergies; see question 44.

44. Do I need to wait to introduce foods with an allergy risk (known as the "Big Eight") to my baby? Or can early introduction of these foods decrease the chance of developing a food allergy?

Current guidance is to feed your baby a wide variety of foods early and often. As long as your pediatrician doesn't recommend waiting, you can feed your baby a tiny amount of any food (other than honey; see question 45) with a consistency and texture that he can handle, starting between 4 and 6 months of age. This includes the "Big Eight" listed here:

- ☐ Milk (if your child is younger than 1 year, offer him yogurt and cheese) (refer to question 48)
- ☐ Eggs (egg white and egg yolk)
- ☐ Peanuts (do not give whole)
- ☐ Tree nuts (such as almonds, do not give whole)
- ☐ Soy
- ☐ Wheat
- ☐ Fish
- ☐ Shellfish (such as shrimp)

Here are some suggestions on how to feed your baby these foods:

- ☐ Add 1 teaspoon of creamy peanut butter or peanut powder to 1 ounce of baby food oatmeal, with extra liquid so it's not too thick and sticky.
- ☐ Puree or fork-mash a hard-boiled egg with a little breast milk or water.
- ☐ Offer plain whole-milk yogurt.
- ☐ Puree wild salmon.
- ☐ Scramble eggs and cut them into tiny pieces for a great first finger food.
- ☐ Offer small pieces of whole-grain O cereal or bread.
- ☐ Spread almond butter thinly on whole-grain bread, and cut it into small pieces.
- ☐ Offer soft-cooked edamame beans (removed from the tough outer shell) and lightly mashed.
- ☐ Give your baby whole milk or reduced-fat (2%) milk after age 1 year. Ask your pediatrician which is best for your child.

Research now shows that feeding your baby potential allergens early and often will get his gut and immune system used to these foods and decrease the chance of developing a food allergy. Although feeding real food is important, it can be challenging to give your baby so many foods so frequently. For this reason, there are commercial products available that incorporate tiny amounts of food proteins. When given regularly (usually a powder to add to food or milk), these products can get your baby's body used to these proteins, so his immune system is less likely to overreact when eating these foods later on.

Toddler Vitamins

The AAP recommends that all children receive 400 IU of vitamin D every day, which can be found in many over-the-counter children's vitamins. Unless your child is drinking 32 ounces a day of vitamin D–fortified milk (and that's a little too much milk!), consider giving your toddler a vitamin supplement. Remember to store the vitamins (as well as all medications and supplements) out of your child's reach. Vitamins can sometimes look and taste like candy, making them appealing to children, but they can be dangerous if not taken as directed.

45. Are there any particular foods to avoid?

There are only 2 recommendations for foods to avoid:

1. **Honey:** *Never give a baby younger than 1 year honey* because of the risk of infant botulism, a deadly disease. Babies, unlike older children and adults, don't have the ability to fight the botulinum toxin sometimes found in honey.
2. **Choking hazards:** Whole nuts, grapes, popcorn, hot dogs, and raw carrots are serious choking hazards, so keep these and other small or hard foods away from infants and toddlers.

46. Should I worry about my toddler's picky eating habits? What can I do?

Between 1 and 5 years of age, children typically experience a slowing of weight gain. They aren't growing as fast as they did during the first year. That means it's normal for children to start eating less at around 12 to 18 months of age. It may seem like they are picky or have a poor appetite. Many will refuse to try new foods or suddenly reject entire food groups that they previously liked. Or your child may want the same food over and over and over. My mom says that I would only eat food with raisins in it until I was 3 years old! Surprisingly, picky eating in a toddler typically won't lead to poor health or nutritional deficiencies.

Don't force your toddler to eat! If you do, mealtime will become the worst time of the day. Sometimes your child's need for control, rather than being picky, causes the problem. So let your child be in charge of what and how much she eats—at least to a certain extent—by offering her a choice between 2 nutritious meals or snacks. Your role as a parent/guardian is to provide and serve the food, and your toddler's role is to choose what she eats. Don't worry, your toddler won't starve herself!

A child's likes and dislikes may change from day to day or month to month. Many children grow well by only eating foods of their favorite color, so be creative—almost every color includes some healthy options.

Remember that a toddler's portion size is about one-third of an adult serving. As a rough guideline for a person of any age, an appropriate portion is usually about the size of that person's palm. For grains, an appropriate amount is about the volume of that person's closed fist. It's also not unusual for children to have 1 good meal, 1 fair meal, and 1 poor meal a day, all of which can ultimately average out to be a fairly decent amount. Offer healthy foods, and let your child eat as much (or as little) as she wants. This will help prevent unnecessary battles from occurring over food.

 When should you worry? Call your pediatrician if you are concerned about your child's growth or weight gain. Don't be afraid to enlist your doctor and/or a pediatric dietician's help in your overall approach to your child's nutrition.

Trial by the Dozens

Studies show that it can take about a dozen tries of a new food item for your child to like it! Keep this in mind as you continue placing those green veggies, like broccoli, on your toddler's tray and show her that you like them too . . . mmm! Eventually, she will start eating them and may grow to like them as well. Try to serve the same foods for the whole family at the dinner table so that she feels included and sees that everyone else is eating their veggies too. Don't give up! It's important to build good habits early. Studies show that the more fruits and veggies eaten as a child, the more fruits and veggies children are likely to eat when they get older.

Dr. Tanya's Tip
Fun and Healthy Eating

Include a variety of food colors on the plate. This is a rough guide for having a good mix of nutrients.

☐ Have your toddler help you in the kitchen by giving him small jobs to do, like handing you ingredients, rinsing fruit, or stirring. He may be more inclined to eat food he helped make. He may make a little mess, but it'll be worth it!

☐ Cut foods (fruit too) into fun shapes by using cookie cutters, or let your toddler help create a fun design or a new dish. This facilitates learning, creativity, and eating!

☐ Use the MyPlate guide: Half of the plate should contain fruits and veggies, one-quarter of the plate is for protein, and one-quarter is for grains.

☐ For more nutrition tips and tricks, a good resource is MyPlate.gov.

Milk (and Other Liquid) Matters

47. How and when do I transition my child from bottle to cup?

Introduce the sippy cup or a cup with a straw around 6 to 9 months of age. Your infant may not take to it immediately, but keep trying. You can start with water to avoid messy spills, but very soon offer breast milk or formula in a cup as well. Once your child has mastered the use of a sippy cup or straw, you can begin to wean him from the bottle, with a goal of having him drink completely out of a cup by 12 to 18 months of age.

If your child is older than 1 year, the transition from bottle to cup can be more challenging, especially if he considers the bottle to be a security or comfort object. You can try gradually weaning him off of the bottle, but often, after around 15 to 18 months of age, it's best to do it all at once. Choose a day, gather up all the bottles, and give them away. If your child is old enough to understand, you can warn him the day before you take the bottles away, explain that you are giving the bottles on his behalf to a younger baby who needs them, and have him help box them up. He may scream and even refuse to drink for a day or two (don't worry, in this short time he won't dehydrate himself), but he'll quickly forget about it and soon take to the sippy cup or cup with a straw. Your ultimate goals are to (a) get him off the bottle by 18 months of age and (b) get him to drink from a regular cup (not a sippy cup) by 2 or 3 years of age.

Dr. Tanya's Tip
Cup That Milk

I see too many parents who only give milk to their children in a bottle and save the sippy cup for water and juice. Then, when it comes time to get rid of the bottle, their child stops drinking milk. But you can avoid this problem. Once you've introduced a sippy cup or a cup with a straw (around 6 to 9 months of age), put breast milk or formula in it. That way, your infant will get used to drinking milk from something other than a breast or bottle. At 1 year of age, when you start giving your child whole or reduced-fat milk, your child will better accept it in a cup, and it will make the transition to drinking milk and weaning your child from the bottle much easier.

48. When can I give my baby regular milk, and how do I introduce it?

You can give your child regular milk, in a cup, at 1 year of age. If your baby is still nursing, you can offer regular milk in a cup and wean her from breast-feeding as you desire. Even if you continue to breast-feed through toddlerhood (hats off to you for sticking with it!), offering occasional sips of milk can help get her used to the taste of cold milk so that when you do eventually wean her off of the breast, she will con-tinue to drink milk. If you are feeding her formula, just switch to regular whole milk. Many 1-year-olds will do fine with the abrupt transition, but if you or she prefers, you can mix the formula with whole milk to transition her to the new, cold taste within a few days. Ideally, your child will drink cold milk straight from the refrigerator in a cup. But if she is currently hooked on a bottle, you can switch her to the taste of regular milk in the bottle first. Then, a few weeks later, you can get rid of the bottle and use a cup.

Experts previously recommended that all 1- to 2-year-olds drink whole milk. They felt that the extra fat was needed for brain development and growth at that age. However, because of the increase in childhood obesity and the high-fat diet of many toddlers, reduced-fat (2%) milk was also deemed fine for this age group. If your toddler is overweight or if there is a family history of obesity, heart disease, or high cholesterol, talk to your pediatrician about giving your toddler 2% milk instead of whole milk at 1 year of age.

For other toddlers, I often stick with whole milk until 18 months of age and then, depending on how they are growing and what else they are eating, switch to 2% milk by 2 years of age. As part of a low-fat, balanced diet, after 2 years of age, most kids (and parents) should transition to low-fat (1%) or nonfat milk. Nonfat milk has essentially the same calcium and nutrients as 1%, 2%, and whole milk, but with each increasing percentage, there is just extra fat (think of pats of butter) stirred in.

49. If my child is allergic to milk, what should I give her to drink and eat?

If your baby is truly allergic to milk (such as getting hives) and has had an allergic reaction to your breast milk, then you should avoid eating any dairy products so there is no milk protein being transferred to your breast milk. Some babies are allergic to milk when they have it directly but are not affected by mom's dairy intake being passed through breast milk.

If you are formula feeding, your doctor may suggest giving your child an extensively hydrolyzed formula that does not contain any milk protein.

If your baby has a nonallergic reaction to milk (such as blood in the stool), you should avoid milk products in your diet as well, at least until your infant outgrows this reaction (around 6 to 12 months of age). You may also need to avoid soy products if elimination of milk products from your diet does not resolve the blood in baby's stool.

If you are formula feeding, your doctor may suggest an amino acid–based formula.

For toddlers and older children who are truly allergic to dairy products (such as getting hives), you should avoid feeding all dairy products, unless your doctor instructs you otherwise.

Talk to your pediatrician or a dietitian about how to ensure that your child is getting all the nutrients needed for proper growth and development. If a child is truly allergic to cow's milk, he is most likely also allergic to milk from other animals, such as goats, because they have similar proteins that could cross-react and lead to an allergic reaction. To ensure that your child gets appropriate nutrition, consider giving her a nondairy milk substitute, such as soy milk, pea protein milk, hemp milk, oat milk, or almond milk, as well as foods high in calcium and vitamin D, such as broccoli, kale, wild salmon, cabbage, salmon, tuna, and fortified cereals.

If your child has a severe allergy, you must check the labels on food packaging to avoid milk products or foods that were produced in factories that also handle milk products. If your child is mildly allergic to milk, your doctor may try giving the child baked products (such as a muffin) in the office, under observation. Remember that some children outgrow their allergies, so the struggle to avoid milk may not last forever.

50. What's the difference between cow, goat, soy, almond, rice, coconut, pea protein, and hemp milk?

There are a lot more differences than many people realize. Cow, soy, goat, and pea protein milk all have around 8 grams of protein per 8-ounce cup. Rice, coconut, and most nut-based milks (like almond) typically have only 1 gram or less of protein per cup. Oat and hemp milk usually have less than 4 grams of protein, but the amount can vary a bit.

Eight grams of protein versus 1 gram of protein is a huge difference for a small child who is drinking 2 cups of milk a day. Milk alternatives also tend to be much lower in calories and other nutrients than dairy milk. Goat's milk lacks folic acid, which can cause anemia in some cases.

To put this in perspective, a toddler who drinks 2 cups of cow's milk a day receives 16 grams of protein and 300 calories; in comparison, a toddler who drinks 2 cups of unfortified almond milk a day receives 2 grams of protein and around 100 calories (depending on the type of almond milk). I have seen many toddlers who aren't gaining enough weight or growing appropriately because their parents didn't make other dietary adjustments when they decided to give their toddler a milk alternative. If your child is allergic to cow's milk or if you choose to give your child a different type of milk, please work with your pediatrician and/or a pediatric dietitian to ensure that your child is getting enough protein, calories, and nutrition for proper growth and development.

51.   One of my toddlers won't eat but loves milk. My other toddler refuses to drink milk. How much milk is too much, and how little is okay?

Many kiddos don't eat because they fill up on liquid calories. Milk (especially if it's whole milk or 2% milk) can be very filling, so it's no wonder that he isn't hungry for food. Limit his milk intake to 16 ounces a day. Serve water with meals and offer milk after he finishes his food. This way, he won't fill up on the milk first.

In most cases, 2 or 3 servings a day of calcium-rich foods are all that your child needs. Toddlers require about 500 mg of calcium daily and can meet these needs by drinking about 2 servings (16 ounces or 2 cups) of milk. (Each cup of milk contains about 300 mg of calcium.) If your child refuses to drink milk, offer 2 to 3 servings of other calcium-rich options, such as yogurt, cheese, green veggies, or orange juice with added calcium (see question 52 for more about juice).

52. When can I give my child fruit juice?

It's actually best if you don't. Your infant or toddler does not need juice. Although 100% fruit juice may have some useful vitamins, juice often contains extra sugar and calories that your child doesn't need. Plus, juice doesn't have the valuable fiber found in fruit. One of the best things you can do for your child's future nutritional health is to get your infant used to drinking water. How many adults do you know who don't like plain water? It's often because they didn't get used to the taste when they were young. Even drinking watered-down juice on a regular basis can get your child in the habit of wanting sweet-tasting beverages. It's best to stick with water and milk whenever possible. If you do choose to give your child juice, keep it under 4 to 6 ounces a day. Treat sweet-tasting drinks like you would a dessert; on special occasions, let your toddler choose juice or another sweet, such as cake. You might be surprised at his choice.

An exception to this recommendation is if your baby is constipated. In such cases, your pediatrician may recommend giving your child small amounts of prune, apple, or pear juice, along with a high-fiber diet, to help with this problem. For more information on constipation, see questions 54 and 55 on pages 96 and 98.

CHAPTER 5

Pooping

Whether we like to admit it or not, a good portion of the first few years of parenting is all about the poop. It begins with that first dark, thick, sticky dirty diaper you change in the hospital and progresses into teaching your child how to get the poop into the potty. There are many colors of poop, the consistency and frequency of the poop may vary, and, oh—how lovely it smells! Poop is definitely on the list of the most common topics parents like to call me about. They often worry their child's poop is too hard, too soft, too much, not enough, or the wrong color. It's rarely "just right." I can't tell you how many emails and texts with photos I've received and poop presents (wrapped in diapers, plastic bags, or even plastic containers) I've been asked to look at. To help you sort out what's right and what might warrant a call to your pediatrician, here's more than you ever thought you would want to know about poop.

Normal Poop

53. What should the poop look like?

While your newborn may already resemble you, her stool won't resemble yours. Baby poop comes in a wide variety of colors and consistencies, and the frequency of pooping varies. Your baby should pass his first stool during the first 24 hours after birth; it will appear thick, sticky, and brownish-black. This is called *meconium*. After the first few days and over the course of the first few weeks, the stools of breastfed babies lighten in color, going from black to brown to green to yellow. They also change in consistency from sticky to seedy to cottage cheese–like to even looser. Breastfed babies will initially produce multiple stools per day, often with every feeding. In contrast, formula-fed babies often have stools that are thicker in consistency and light brown. Unlike breastfed babies, formula-fed babies generally produce stool once per day on average.

As infants grow, their stool pattern tends to slow down. Some may poop many times a day, while others poop every few days. The color of the poop may range from yellow to brown, with a green one thrown in every so often for added color. Yes, green stools may be quite normal!

With an increase in solid food intake, toddler stools typically look (and smell) more like adult stools. Some variation in color and consistency is normal, often depending on what children eat and drink. If you find a neon green surprise in your toddler's diaper, it may be the dye in the juice your toddler is drinking—just one more reason to give your toddler water instead!

The following bullets can help you gauge whether your child is constipated.

- ☐ Type 1: Painful, very thick, dense, heavy rocks/ pebbles/pellets, hard to push out
- ☐ Type 2: Hard to push out initially, clumped-together pebbles
- ☐ Type 3: Soft and easy to push out in log shapes
- ☐ Type 4: Super soft, semisolid, comes out easily and/or explosively
- ☐ Type 5: Liquid, runs out, hard to control

Stool types 1 and 2 suggest constipation, which means your child may need more fiber and fluids (like water). Type 3 is normal and easy to pass. Types 4 and 5 may be a sign of too much juice, illness, or other disease process that is causing soft stools and/or diarrhea. The goal is for most stools to look like type 3. There will always be some daily variation due to diet, water intake, and activity, so don't be alarmed if just 1 or 2 stools are different types. Look for consistent patterns.

 Although variation in stool color is normal, some colors do warrant further investigation. If your child starts to have black stools after the first few days following birth, or if they are red or bloody, white, chalky, or clay colored, call your pediatrician and bring in a stool sample to be checked out.

Constipation

54. My baby hasn't pooped for 3 days. What should I do?

Believe it or not, this is one of the more common questions pediatricians hear. In the first few weeks after birth, your newborn really should poop every day; if not, let your pediatrician know. As infants grow, they usually poop less than they did as a newborn, and some may poop only once a week. Although less frequent pooping can be normal, it's possible that your baby isn't drinking enough to produce frequent poop. Rarely, there could be something hindering the stool from coming out, such as a condition called *Hirschsprung disease,* in which the end of the intestines or the anus isn't working properly.

After learning that all of your baby's parts are working well—producing at least 1 stool before going home from the hospital and logging a few good weeks of eating and pooping regularly—it is normal for a breastfed baby to produce stool anywhere from roughly once every 5 days up to 11 times a day. At about 2 months of age, your baby's pooping pattern may change, usually becoming less frequent. Formula-fed babies tend to poop less often than breastfed babies. As long as your baby is acting fine and drinking enough breast milk or formula, and as long as the stool itself isn't too hard, just wait. He will eventually poop.

Generally speaking, the answer is . . . don't worry! As infants grow, they usually poop less than they did

as a newborn, and some may poop only once a week
(how nice for those lucky few parents). In addition,
they may push, grunt, and strain—all in the name of
a poop. Their faces may also turn as red as a tomato.
As long as what comes out is soft, these behaviors
are fine. Remember that your baby is learning how to
poop and has to develop the proper coordination to
make it happen. So if your infant is drinking and eating well (if he is already eating solid food) and if the
stool isn't too hard, give him some time to let it come
out. If the stool is large and hard or looks like small
rocks, or if your baby hasn't pooped for a few days
and is very uncomfortable, try giving him an ounce or
two of water, prune juice, or pureed baby food prunes
to help soften the stool and make it easier for him to
push out. If any of these options don't help after a few
days, call your pediatrician; he or she may suggest a
suppository or, rarely, medication to help.

 Call your pediatrician if you have any concerns, including the
following:

- ☐ Your baby's belly seems to be swollen or distended.
- ☐ Your baby starts vomiting.
- ☐ Your baby develops a fever.
- ☐ Your baby is tired and not interested in feeding.

If your otherwise healthy newborn isn't producing stool at
least once a day for the first few weeks after birth or, after
that, if your baby has gone an entire week without pooping,
let your pediatrician know.

Dr. Tanya's Tip
Palatable Prunes

If your constipated baby won't drink prune juice or water, mix it with some breast milk or formula and he'll be more likely to take it. I know it sounds strange, but babies love prune juice mixed with breast milk! Once your infant is eating solid food, try feeding him pureed baby prunes. Some babies do well if they are given a little pureed prune every morning for breakfast by itself or mixed into cereal, other fruit, or yogurt. For toddlers who feed themselves, try giving them diced prunes, cut into tiny pieces. Prunes are sweet, and most babies and toddlers will quickly grow to like the taste. Getting infants and toddlers used to eating prunes on a regular basis is a healthy habit that will easily prevent and/or treat many tummy aches and constipation issues. If your infant or toddler is still having issues with producing stools, check in with your pediatrician to make sure nothing else is needed.

55. My toddler has a tendency to become constipated. What can I give her to soften her stools and prevent this from happening again?

Constipation is common in toddlers and can cause endless problems. If pooping hurts, they won't do it. So they hold it in, which makes it hurt even more. This can also lead to diarrhea or leakage of stool around the harder stool that your toddler has not yet eliminated. All of this can also really interfere with potty training (see question 142, on page 245). Correcting and preventing constipation are very important, no matter how old your kids are.

Establishing regular bowel movements in infancy and toddlerhood can help prevent a lifetime of straining and toilet problems. Things you can do to encourage a pattern of regular pooping include the following:

☐ Water should always be the first drink of choice after breast milk or formula. Drinking water helps stool pass through the intestines.

☐ Give your child high-fiber foods, such as leafy green vegetables, broccoli, cauliflower, peas, plums and prunes, raisins, oatmeal, and whole-grain cereals and bread. When buying packaged foods, always check the label for the amount of fiber (3 grams or more is best).

☐ Avoid giving your child too many constipating foods, such as bananas, rice, and cereals and breads that are not high in fiber, if you are not balancing these foods with other fiber-rich components of a regular, healthy diet.

☐ Set up a regular toilet routine and make it fun—generally, using the toilet should happen after every meal. This way, you will take advantage of the body's natural reflex to poop after a meal.

☐ Promote physical activity! This is generally not hard for busy toddlers and children, but as children spend more time with electronic devices, it is important to ensure that they spend lots of time on the move every day.

To help your child with constipation when it does arise, here are some tips:

☐ Some fruits are natural laxatives, including prunes, plums, cherries, apricots, pears, and grapes. Some fruit juices, such as prune juice, apple juice, apricot nectar, and pear nectar, also can help with constipation. I find that prune juice seems to work the best. If your child won't drink prune juice (make sure you tell her how yummy it is!), mix 1 part prune juice with 2 parts apple juice. Apple juice works too, but some kids need 2 to 3 cups of it a day (not watered down), which is a lot of sugar. Drinking plenty of water every day will help with constipation as well.

☐ Be sure to include fiber in your family's daily diet. If you read labels, you'll be surprised by the high number of good-tasting, high-fiber options. High-fiber whole-wheat bread, tortillas, and soft granola bars are good choices. Look for high-fiber crackers—eating a few of these a day can keep many previously constipated preschoolers regular. If dietary changes aren't working well enough, talk to your pediatrician about a plan to help soften your toddler's stools. Your child may benefit from a special diet or trying an over-the-counter medication.

Diarrhea

56. Why does my child get horrible diarrhea almost every winter?

Rotavirus was the most common infectious cause of diarrhea in children until the vaccine came out (yay!), and now norovirus tops the charts as the most common cause of infectious diarrhea at all ages. Both strike most often during the winter months; many parents refer to this type of infection as the "stomach flu," even though there's no relation between these viruses and influenza, which causes cough and high fever.

The typical course is fever and vomiting for a few days, often followed by green, foul-smelling, watery diarrhea for a week or sometimes even longer. Older children and adults (who have stronger immune systems) may get lucky and only have mild symptoms, but many younger children can have serious vomiting and diarrhea. Young children in particular are more likely to be hospitalized from dehydration caused by these viruses. It can spread like wildfire throughout child care centers and preschools, where children are in close contact with each other and have an increased risk of spreading and sharing germs. How do you reduce your family's chances of catching it? Wash your hands often and properly and teach your children to do the same.

57. What should I give my child when he has diarrhea?

The most important thing is to give your child plenty of liquids. This is often easier said than done, especially when everything is coming out of the other end so quickly. If your child is also vomiting, keeping him hydrated can be even more challenging (see question 58, on page 104).

Newborns and young infants with diarrhea can easily become dehydrated, so it's particularly important to call your pediatrician to discuss what to do and determine the cause of the diarrhea. Continue giving your newborn breast milk or formula unless your doctor directs you to stop. The pediatrician may recommend increasing your baby's fluid intake, giving your baby an oral rehydration fluid (such as Pedialyte), or changing your baby's formula to a lactose-free version until the diarrhea eases up. Your doctor may also want to examine and weigh your newborn every day or every few days to make sure he isn't losing weight. If your newborn has a fever with diarrhea, he should be evaluated immediately by your pediatrician or another physician to make sure there is not a more serious infection going on.

Your older infant or toddler may not feel like consuming much solid food while he is sick. That's okay, as long as he continues drinking fluids. If your child is older than 1 year and is drinking regular milk that seems to make the diarrhea worse, you may want to try lactose-free milk for a few days. Electrolyte replacement drinks can also help keep kids hydrated. When he does feel like eating, keep it simple initially with cereal, bananas, mashed potatoes, applesauce, bread, and rice and then advance to his regular diet as tolerated. Avoid giving him juice or sugary beverages if possible, as this may worsen the diarrhea. Because the ultimate goal is to stay hydrated, if juice is absolutely the only thing your infant or toddler will drink, try a juice with lower sugar content and water it down if you can.

For all ages: In addition to the hassle of managing diarrhea, help prevent an irritating and potentially painful diaper rash by coating your little one's bottom at every diaper change with a diaper cream that contains zinc oxide. Despite your best efforts, a rash may still develop. If this is the case, use wipes made mainly with water or wash her bottom gently in the sink after a bowel movement, and continue to coat the skin well with a protective layer of diaper cream or ointment; for further advice, refer to question 102 on page 173.

 Call your doctor if any of the following occurs:

- ☐ Your child refuses to drink fluids.
- ☐ The diarrhea contains blood or excessive mucus.
- ☐ Your child has fewer wet diapers than usual.
- ☐ The diarrhea lasts for more than 2 weeks.
- ☐ Your infant or toddler is producing more than 8 stools per day.

58. How do I know if my child is dehydrated?

Dehydration is one of the most worrisome complications of an otherwise ordinary case of diarrhea. Paying attention to a few details will help you recognize the signs of dehydration.

If any of the following signs are present, call your pediatrician and seek medical attention.

- ☐ **Urine output:** Your child may be urinating less as his body is trying to hold onto water. As a rule of thumb, he should still have at least 3 wet diapers in a 24-hour period.
- ☐ **Energy:** Most children can feel pretty tired when they have diarrhea, and they may sleep more than usual. However, they should be arousable. If you find that it is difficult to awaken your child from sleep or your child seems confused, these are signs that she may need additional help with staying hydrated, such as receiving medication to help keep fluids down or intravenous fluids.
- ☐ **Change in appearance:** If your child has sunken eyes, no tears when crying, and a dry mouth or lips, these are all signs of dehydration.
- ☐ **Refusal to drink anything:** If your child is unwilling to take even sips of water or ice chips over the course of multiple hours, she may need additional help with staying hydrated, such as being given intravenous fluids.

59. After a few days of taking an antibiotic for an illness, my child started having loose stools. Is this an allergy? Should I stop giving her the medicine?

Loose stools are not caused by an allergic reaction to the medicine. Diarrhea and mild abdominal pain are 2 of the most common side effects of antibiotics. In addition, the loose stools may just be part of the original illness. As long as you keep your child hydrated by giving her plenty of fluids, the loose stools shouldn't cause any harm (although you may have to treat a diaper rash). The diarrhea will likely stop soon after the course of antibiotics is completed and the illness is over. Do not stop giving your child the antibiotic without calling your pediatrician first.

It's a good idea to give your child probiotics daily (even when not being treated with antibiotics, because of the benefits of good gut bacteria) to help replace the good gut bacteria that antibiotics can wipe out. You can start giving your child a probiotic (chewable, powder, or liquid) or yogurt (or other drink) with live cultures and probiotics while she is still taking the antibiotic—just give her the probiotic a few hours before or after taking the antibiotic. Continue giving her probiotics for at least a week or two after completing the antibiotic course.

Call your pediatrician if there is any vomiting or blood in the stool, if there are more than 8 loose stools a day, or if the diarrhea persists after the medication is stopped. In addition, if a fever persists for more than 2 to 3 days after starting antibiotic treatment, see your pediatrician to find out if the initial infection is resolving or if there needs to be a change in the treatment plan.

CHAPTER 6

Stomachaches and Vomiting

There's nothing quite as distinct as the smell of my office after a child with a stomach virus has visited. Fortunately, not all stomachaches are associated with the upheaval of stomach contents. In fact, complaints of tummy pain are fairly common, from toddler age on up. Differentiating between a complaint that is serious and one that is just due to too many snacks can be challenging, especially when there are tears involved. Although complaints of pain from your child should not be taken lightly, this chapter will provide some basic guidelines to help you figure out when you should worry and when you can relax.

Tummy Troubles

60. My toddler often complains of a tummy ache. It comes and goes, but the pain is not severe. What should I do?

As long as the pain isn't severe, worsening, or interfering with activity, you can take a moment to assess the situation. There are several questions that your pediatrician may ask, so it can be quite helpful to gather the information he or she will need ahead of time to help figure out what's causing the pain. Here are some of the many questions that your pediatrician may ask when you call:

- ☐ How long has the pain been present? Has it been days, weeks, or months?
- ☐ How bad is the pain? Does it make your child cry?
- ☐ Where is the pain? Is it around the belly button or the lower right belly?
- ☐ How long does the pain last? Does anything seem to make it better or worse?
- ☐ Is there any fever, vomiting, or diarrhea?
- ☐ Does the pain wake your toddler up at night or interfere with activity?
- ☐ Does the pain occur only on preschool days or during a particular time of day?
- ☐ How is your child's appetite?
- ☐ Is the pain related to any specific food or drink, such as milk products? Or is the pain better or worse after your child eats?

- [ ] Is your toddler potty trained? Does the pain occur only when she needs to poop?
- [ ] Does your child poop every day? Is the stool hard or soft? Is it big or small? Is there any blood in the stool?
- [ ] Has there been any recent social or family stress or a change in environment?
- [ ] Is there any family history of stomach or intestinal diseases or issues?
- [ ] Has there been any recent travel or exposure to pets?

It is often useful to keep a diary in the days leading up to your office visit (and sometimes even longer) and to bring your notes with you to your appointment. The diary should include what your child eats and drinks, when the pain occurs, what she is doing at the time the pain occurs, how long it lasts, and, most importantly, how often she poops and what it looks like. Also, let the doctor's office know exactly why you are coming in (eg, your child has experienced stomachaches on and off for 3 months) so they can schedule extra time for the appointment, if needed.

Soothing Stomach Cramps

There is no perfect way to help soothe a crampy tummy. Some parents find that giving their child simethicone or other infant gas drops may help soothe their gassy baby. For older infants and toddlers, having a warm bath and taking sips of cool chamomile or peppermint tea may bring some relief. What caused the tummy ache? It may be gas, constipation, or a bit of an upset stomach. It may also be the first sign of a developing stomach virus or a "stomach bug" (sometimes called the *"stomach flu"*), which means that vomiting and diarrhea will usually follow. Consult your doctor for the following reasons:

- ☐ Your child's symptoms persist.
- ☐ The symptoms are severe.
- ☐ Your child develops a fever.
- ☐ Your child doesn't want to eat or drink.
- ☐ Your child isn't acting well.

61. My child has a bad stomachache. When should I worry?

Infants and toddlers often can't tell you that their tummy hurts, so it can take some detective work on your part to figure out when you really need to call your pediatrician and have your child evaluated. The following signs and symptoms should be taken seriously because they may indicate a more pressing medical issue.

Call your pediatrician or schedule an appointment right away if any of the following is true:

- ☐ Your child looks sick.
- ☐ Your child's pain is severe (especially if it's on the lower right side of the abdomen).
- ☐ Your child's pain is worsening.

- ☐ Your child's pain is constant for more than 2 hours.
- ☐ Your child has a swollen, distended, or tender belly.
- ☐ Your child has no interest in eating her favorite food.
- ☐ Your child has persistent or projectile vomiting.
- ☐ Your child has persistent diarrhea.
- ☐ Your child's poop is bloody or dark or looks like grape jelly.
- ☐ Your toddler can't jump up and down without feeling pain.
- ☐ Your toddler can't walk because of the pain or walks hunched over.
- ☐ Your child has pain with urination or decreased urination (fewer than 3 times per day).
- ☐ Your child has excruciating pain that comes and goes multiple times a day.

62. How do I know if my child's tummy ache is appendicitis?

Even doctors sometimes have a tough time diagnosing appendicitis, especially in young children, which is one of the reasons why a stomachache associated with any of the symptoms listed in the previous question should be evaluated right away. Typically, the signs and symptoms of appendicitis are tummy pain that starts around the belly button and, over several hours, moves to the lower right part of the belly. A child will cry or say it hurts when that area is pushed on. In addition, a child may vomit, have a fever, and not want to eat a favorite food if offered. Asking a toddler to jump can provide another clue. If it's appendicitis, most people—toddlers and adults alike—won't jump because it hurts when they do.

 Infants and toddlers with appendicitis don't always exhibit the expected signs and symptoms, especially if they are younger than 2 years old. Call your pediatrician if your child has any of the symptoms listed under question 61 or if you are concerned about appendicitis. The doctor will need to examine your child and may order some tests, including ultrasonography or a computed tomographic (CT) scan to look for appendicitis.

63. Sometimes I notice a bulge in my child's belly. Is this normal? Could it be a hernia?

When children are crying intensely, they can swallow a lot of air. This can cause their stomachs to look distended. If a specific area is bulging (not the entire belly), this might be concerning for a hernia. Hernias develop when there is an opening in the abdominal wall that allows the contents to squeeze through (most often the intestines). Pressure within the abdomen, which can occur with crying, coughing, or vomiting, can cause these contents to protrude further. Lying down reduces the pressure and often makes the bulge disappear. Umbilical and inguinal hernias are the most common types of abdominal hernias in children.

Umbilical hernias (or "outie" belly buttons, as they're more commonly called) are usually not worrisome in children. The abdominal muscles come together as a baby grows, and the hernia usually goes away by age 2 to 4 years. If the hernia is quite large and not getting smaller with time, you can talk to your pediatrician about having a pediatric surgeon perform a small corrective surgery.

Inguinal hernias appear as bulges in the lower abdomen or groin region and occur more commonly in boys. With an inguinal hernia, you may notice a difference in the size of your son's testicles. Inguinal hernias can occur on both sides of the abdomen. If you observe these symptoms, let your pediatrician know, and she will refer you to a surgeon for evaluation and treatment.

In general, having a hernia is not an emergency situation if the bulge is painless and your child is eating well.

 If your child is in severe pain or is vomiting, however, call your pediatrician or go to the emergency department right away. If these symptoms persist, emergency surgery may be needed to fix the hernia.

Vomiting and Dehydration

64. What should I give my child when he is vomiting?

More often than not, what may seem to be *newborn* vomiting is actually just a lot of spit-up, caused by taking in too much fluid too quickly, or reflux. (For more information about reflux, see question 40.) However, true vomiting in a newborn *does* need to be evaluated, as it could be a sign of something more serious or lead to significant dehydration. Your pediatrician may recommend giving your newborn a little less fluid at the next feeding to see if it stays down. However, if the vomiting persists, this warrants a trip to your pediatrician's office or even the emergency department if your doctor's office is closed.

 If your **newborn's** vomit becomes projectile (shoots a few feet across the room), is forceful, happens more than a few times, or occurs after 2 or more feedings in a row, that's a good reason to call the pediatrician. In addition, if the vomit contains any bright red blood or dark brown "coffee ground" material or if you have any other questions or concerns, call your pediatrician immediately or go to the emergency department.

When *an older infant or a toddler* is actively vomiting, it's best to hold off on giving him anything to eat or drink. Once the vomiting seems to have stopped, try giving him very small amounts of clear fluids frequently. Start with 1 teaspoon of fluid every 10 minutes. If that stays down for an hour or so, you can slowly increase the amount you give him. Your pediatrician may recommend that you start with a clear electrolyte solution (such as Pedialyte). After several hours without further vomiting, your pediatrician may advise you to return to giving your child small amounts of milk (breast milk, formula, or cow's milk) or whatever your child likes to drink for a few feedings before increasing slowly to the usual amounts. Many parents make the mistake of letting their thirsty child drink a few ounces at once, but with an uneasy stomach, it will all come back up. It's best to avoid solids and stick with liquids for several hours after the vomiting has subsided. When you do introduce solids, go very slowly. Start small and simply, such as giving your child 1 spoonful of oatmeal or 1 cracker, and then wait about 30 minutes to see what happens.

 For older infants and toddlers, call your pediatrician if you have any of the following concerns:

- ☐ Your older infant or toddler is unable to keep even small amounts of fluids down.
- ☐ Your child's vomiting persists for more than a few hours.
- ☐ There is bright red blood or dark brown "coffee ground" material in your child's vomit.
- ☐ The vomit is bright green or yellow.
- ☐ Your child shows signs of dehydration (see question 65).

Dr. Tanya's Tip

"Recipe" for Keeping Fluids Down in Toddlers

To avoid ending up in the hospital with your child having to receive intravenous fluids, consider this "recipe" of steps to take with toddlers who are vomiting. If you are going through the steps and vomiting reoccurs, stop and go back one step in the recipe. If vomiting *continues*, it's important to call your pediatrician or go to the emergency department. With infants, it's best to touch base with your pediatrician before trying this or any other hydration plan. As with all recipes (even those from Grandma's kitchen), there may be similar versions that yield good results. Ultimately, the goal is to start small and increase the amount as tolerated so that your child can keep 4 to 8 ounces of fluids down over several hours.

Hour 1:   Give your child nothing to drink.

Hour 2:   Give 1 teaspoon of clear electrolyte solution every 10 minutes.

Hour 3:   Give 2 teaspoons of clear electrolyte solution every 15 minutes.

Hour 4:   Give 0.5 ounce of clear electrolyte solution every 20 minutes.

Hour 5:   Give 1 ounce of clear electrolyte solution every 30 minutes.

Hour 6:   Very slowly resume a normal fluid intake. (Giving your child formula or breast milk is usually fine.)

65.   What is dehydration, and when do I need to worry about it?

Dehydration is always a concern with sick children. It happens when infants and young children aren't drinking enough fluids or are vomiting, with or without diarrhea, since they can easily and quickly become dehydrated this way. Dehydration can manifest in a variety of ways but usually appears as fewer wet diapers, less energy, dry lips or tongue, and more severe signs, as noted in the following paragraphs.

To prevent dehydration when your child is not feeling well, give her small amounts of fluids frequently—as long as she can keep the fluids down.

 Newborns can become dehydrated very quickly. Don't wait until the signs of dehydration (as specified here for infants and toddlers) are present to get help. If a newborn is vomiting, drinking less than usual, or having fewer wet or dirty diapers than normal, call your pediatrician.

Call your pediatrician if your child is not keeping even small amounts of fluids down, if vomiting persists for more than a few hours, if diarrhea persists for more than a few days, or if there are any signs of dehydration, such as fewer wet diapers or less urine being produced, lack of energy or more tiredness than usual, no tears when your child cries, dry lips and tongue, a sunken fontanelle (the soft spot on top of the head), irritability, or sunken eyes.

CHAPTER 7

Fever

M any parents panic when their child feels warm. "Could it be? Oh no, it's a fever! Call the doctor!" A fever isn't a disease itself—just a symptom or, rather, a byproduct of an illness. Fever is actually helpful; it is your body's attempt to "turn up the heat" on germs, making your body a very uncomfortable place for these unwanted houseguests. If your baby is younger than 3 months, it may be appropriate to worry and it is definitely appropriate to call your pediatrician—no matter what the time. As long as your child is older than 3 months and has received his first set of vaccines, though, the thermometer reading may not make much of a difference. What actually matters is how your child is acting (interacting, eating, and sleeping, in particular) and what other symptoms your child has (such as coughing or vomiting). The questions in this chapter contain information and guidelines about fever and when you should call your pediatrician. I know I've said it before, but it really is true—as a parent, you know your child best, so if you feel something is wrong, never hesitate to call at any time.

Who, What, When, Where, Why, and How?

What Is a Fever?

Normal body temperature is around 98.6°F (37°C), plus or minus 1°F (0.6°C), and varies throughout the day. Everyone's internal thermostat is a little bit different, so in general, a range from 97.6°F (36.4°C) to 100.3°F (37.9°C) is considered normal. A temperature of 100.4°F (38°C) or higher, obtained rectally, is considered a fever.

66. What causes a fever? When do I need to call the doctor?

A fever is usually caused by infections from viruses (such as a cold virus or the flu) or bacteria (such as strep throat or some ear infections). Remember, the fever itself is not the disease, only a sign that the body's defenses are trying to fight an infection.

 Whatever your child's age, some symptoms that occur along with a fever warrant a more urgent call to your pediatrician, because they may indicate a more serious illness or situation developing. Call your doctor if your little one has a fever and any of the following symptoms:

☐ Refusal or inability to drink fluids
☐ Continuous crying
☐ Irritability after lowering the fever temperature
    with appropriate medication
☐ Difficulty waking up
☐ Confusion
☐ Rash
☐ Stiff neck
☐ Trouble breathing or rapid breathing
☐ Persistent vomiting
☐ Diarrhea
☐ Seizure

You should also call your doctor if a fever persists for more than 3 days. If the fever lasts for longer than 4 or 5 days, your child should be evaluated by a doctor, even if the fever is not accompanied by any of the worrisome symptoms described here. If you think your child really looks sick or if you are worried about something in particular, always call your doctor, regardless of your child's temperature.

The definition of fever for each age does vary slightly among pediatricians, but here are some general guidelines.

Infant younger than 3 months: Call your pediatrician immediately if your baby has a temperature of *100.4°F (38°C) or higher—even if your baby looks well.* If the pediatrician can't be reached, go straight to the emergency department.

Infant older than 3 months: If your infant has a temperature above 102°F (39°C), call your pediatrician. The doctor will likely ask you about other symptoms (eg, cough, cold, vomiting, diarrhea) and how your child is acting overall to help determine if you need to bring him in for an evaluation or if you can wait and watch him at home for a few days.

Infants and toddlers older than 6 months: If your child has a temperature of 104°F (40°C) or higher, this warrants a call to the pediatrician's office (you'll probably be calling before you read this anyway). Otherwise, the child can be watched at home as long as he is alert, interacting, and drinking fluids. If the symptoms aren't improving in 2 or 3 days or if they are worsening, see your pediatrician.

67. How often do I need to take my child's temperature, and what's the best way?

There is really no need to randomly check your child's temperature. If she feels unusually warm, is not eating well, or is irritable or overly sleepy, use a thermometer to check for a fever.

Obtaining a rectal temperature is the most accurate and preferred method for a newborn. Although the idea may seem uncomfortable to you, it won't hurt your baby. Just coat the end of the thermometer with a lubricant (such as water-based K-Y Jelly or petroleum jelly) and insert the thermometer about half an inch into your baby's rectum (follow the instructions for your particular thermometer). Digital thermometers provide a quick, fairly accurate reading—within a minute, you'll know your baby's temperature. If the thermometer reads 100.4°F (38°C) or higher, your newborn has a fever, which may sometimes indicate a serious infection. Although most newborn fevers are not serious, little ones can get very sick very quickly and should be evaluated as soon as possible, even if it means a trip to the emergency department in the middle of the night!

Although rectal temperatures are most accurate, let's be practical. Your older infant or toddler is less likely to lie still long enough for you to get a good reading. For older infants and toddlers, a digital thermometer held under the arm, an ear thermometer, or a temporal artery (forehead) thermometer is fine. If the thermometer reads 100.4°F (38°C) or higher, it's best to double-check the temperature rectally before calling your pediatrician, especially with an infant. In contrast to what you may have heard in the past, there is no need to add or subtract a degree depending on where and how you obtained the temperature; just let your pediatrician know how the temperature was measured and how your child is acting.

 Immediately call your pediatrician if your baby is younger than 3 months and has a temperature of 100.4°F (38°C) or higher. If you have any concerns that your newborn or young infant might be sick—even in the absence of a fever—call your pediatrician.

Fever Feelings

All kids (and most adults too) can feel and act miserable when they have a fever, no matter what other symptoms they have. What's important is how they are feeling when the fever comes down. If they are playing and running around the house, or feel and look better after a dose of fever-reducing medication, that's a good sign that they are probably not seriously ill.

 If your child is still not acting well once the fever comes down, call your pediatrician.

68. My child has a fever, without any other symptoms. Do I need to take her to the doctor? When should I worry?

For infants older than 3 months and toddlers, as long as they are acting well, you can observe them for a few days. With some viral infections, such as roseola (see chapter 10, Skin), children can have a fever without any other symptoms for 2 or 3 days. The fever will go away and then there may be a rash (don't worry, it's not dangerous). With most other illnesses, you will see some additional symptoms (eg, cough, runny nose, diarrhea) within 24 hours of the fever. Viral fevers can easily last for up to 4 or 5 days, but longer than that may mean there is another infection going on that may require treatment.

If your baby is younger than 3 months and has a temperature of 100.4°F (38°C) or higher, immediately call your
pediatrician. Newborns and young infants do not always
show signs of illness besides having a fever, and they can get
sick very quickly, so it's important not to wait.

It's also important to check with your pediatrician before
giving your newborn any fever-reducing medication.

If your infant is older than 3 months and has had a fever
for more than 3 or 4 days without any other symptoms, call
your pediatrician. The doctor will want to examine her and
may check her urine and even blood to make sure there isn't an
infection hiding somewhere that hasn't yet presented itself.

69. My daughter has a fever. Do I need to give her medicine?

Remember that a fever is just a sign that your child's
body is fighting an infection. The reason your doctor
may recommend medicine to reduce a fever is so that
your child may feel more comfortable (and therefore
you will as well). It is very important that your child
continues to drink fluids (eating popsicles and Jell-O
works too) to help avoid dehydration that can occur
with a fever. However, if she is so miserable with
a fever that she cannot drink, then medicine may
help. However, if she's acting well and drinking fluids
despite having a higher-than-normal temperature,
you don't have to give her medicine; the fever itself
isn't dangerous, can help fight infection, and will
more than likely go away with some time.

Medication such as acetaminophen (Tylenol) or ibuprofen (Motrin or Advil) can be given in appropriate doses to reduce the fever. *Do not give your child aspirin* because it can cause Reye syndrome, a serious disease that can damage the brain and liver. Ibuprofen (only for infants older than 6 months) lasts 6 to 8 hours, while acetaminophen lasts 4 to 6 hours. Both are dosed by weight, so check with your pediatrician or pharmacist if you are not sure about the correct dose for your child. To help avoid an accidental overdose, read package labels very carefully and always use the dropper or medicine cup that came with the specific medication you are giving. Measuring medicine in milliliters (mL) is always more accurate than teaspoons.

Note: Infants' and children's formulations of ibuprofen have different concentrations (see the following dosing charts). Acetaminophen concentration is the same for infants' and children's formulations.

 For older infants and toddlers, call your pediatrician if your child is not acting well when his temperature comes down or if you find yourself needing to give these medications for more than 4 days.

Acetaminophen (Tylenol) Dosing Chart		
Child's Weight/ Approximate Age	Infant's Suspension Liquid (160 mg/5 mL)	Children's Suspension Liquid (160 mg/5 mL)
6-11 lb/0-5 mo	1.25 mL	1.25 mL
12-17 lb/6-11 mo	2.5 mL	2.5 mL
18-23 lb/12-23 mo	3.75 mL	3.75 mL
24-35 lb/2-3 y	5 mL	5 mL

Acetaminophen can be given every 4 to 6 hours as needed, up to 5 times a day.

Ibuprofen (Motrin or Advil) Dosing Chart		
Child's Weight/ Approximate Age	Infant's Concentrated Drops (50 mg/1.25 mL)	Children's Suspension Liquid (100 mg/5 mL)
6–11 lb/0–5 mo	Do not use	Do not use
12–17 lb/6–11 mo	1.25 mL	2.5 mL
18–23 lb/12–23 mo	1.875 mL (1.25 mL + 0.625 mL)	3.75 mL
24–35 lb/2–3 y	2.50 mL (1.25 mL + 1.25 mL)	5 mL

Ibuprofen can be given every 6 to 8 hours as needed, up to 4 times a day.

Dr. Tanya's Tip
Avoid Medication Mistakes

☐ Read package labels very carefully.

☐ Always use the dropper or medicine cup that comes with the specific medication you are giving.

☐ Call your pediatrician if you are unsure about the appropriate dose for your child.

☐ Keep a written log of the time the medication is given and the amount of medication given.

☐ Do not give more than one medication at a time without consulting your physician.

☐ Keep all medications safely out of your child's reach.

☐ Make sure all caregivers are aware of the medication dose and when it needs to be given.

70. I just gave my child a fever reducer, but she still has a fever. Now what can I do?

If your child is acting better after taking a fever reducer (she is smiling and drinking fluids), but she still has a fever, it's usually okay. Your child's behavior is often more important than the number on the thermometer. You can check the dose with your pediatrician (or read the chart in the previous question) to make sure you gave your child enough medication, as kids are constantly growing and their dose increases as they gain weight. Giving your child plenty of fluids and using the techniques described in the following answer can also help bring the fever down. It's important to make sure you don't accidentally double up on medication with the same active ingredient (such as 2 types of fever reducers that both contain acetaminophen). Giving multiple medications with acetaminophen may result in serious liver toxicity. Likewise, overdosing with ibuprofen may result in serious toxicity.

 Check with your pediatrician before giving your newborn any fever-reducing medication. Again, if your baby is younger than 3 months and has a fever, always call your doctor immediately or go to the emergency department.

Call your pediatrician if your infant or toddler isn't looking well after taking a dose of fever reducer. There may be something more serious going on than a simple viral infection, and your pediatrician may want to have your child evaluated.

71. What can I do to help my child with a fever, besides giving him medicine?

Just like playing out in the hot sun, being warm from a fever causes your child to sweat and lose more water through his skin than he usually would. To keep up with his water loss, it is important for him to drink lots of fluids (eg, water, breast milk or formula, or an electrolyte solution) to avoid becoming dehydrated. Cool liquids will feel good and help replace needed fluids in his body. Even if your child does not feel like eating food, he should continue to drink to prevent him from using up all of his body's water.

If your baby has a fever, be careful not to wrap him in too many layers. Wrapping your baby in lots of layers when he has a fever can cause his temperature to go higher, since he is too young to undress himself or tell you that he feels warm. Babies are very sensitive to overheating and can quickly become too hot when bundled tightly in the heat or during a fever.

For older children with a fever, removing layers of clothing can also be helpful because it will enable them to lose heat through the skin. For babies, this means dressing them in 1 layer of light clothing and wrapping them in a single light blanket. For older children, you can remove blankets or clothing. There are cool gel pads created for kids to wear. Sponging your child's skin with lukewarm (never cold) water may also help decrease the fever and make him feel better. Stop sponging your child or use warmer water if he becomes cold or begins to shiver.

Other Fever Factors

72. Can teething cause a fever?

Although many parents sometimes notice that their child feels warm or has a low-grade fever, teething does not actually cause a true fever (a temperature higher than 100.4°F or 38°C). If your teething infant does have a fever, it is probably due to something else—possibly a cold or other illness that hasn't presented itself yet. Teething usually isn't fun, even without a fever, as it can cause quite a bit of drool and fussiness as the teeth poke their way through sensitive gums—ouch! For infants (or even toddlers) who seem to be bothered by teething, it may help to give them an appropriate dose of acetaminophen, along with a cool teething ring from the refrigerator to chew on. You can also gently massage your baby's gums with your clean fingertip (or wear clean gloves), which may be soothing. Frozen popsicles or a damp washcloth twisted and frozen also works well for toddlers.

Don't freeze teething rings since making them too cold can injure a baby's gums.

Don't use numbing gels that contain benzocaine, as they are not recommended for babies.

Depending on how high your infant's temperature is and how she is acting, you can observe your teething child for a day or two or call your pediatrician for advice.

73. My child had his shots today. Now he has a fever. Should I worry?

Vaccines are important because they can protect your child from potentially dangerous and deadly diseases. Vaccines are safe, and severe reactions are very rare. Mild reactions to vaccines may occur, such as a low-grade fever and fussiness, but fortunately they do not last long. There may be some swelling, redness, and discomfort where the shot was given. Another common side effect is a pea-sized lump under the skin at the site of the injection. This is not dangerous and will resolve over the next few weeks.

Some infants and toddlers will develop a fever after receiving their immunizations. Having a mild fever without any other symptoms is not dangerous. You may give an appropriate dose of infant acetaminophen for a temperature above 100.4°F (38°C) if your infant seems cranky. Your pediatrician may recommend giving your child a dose of acetaminophen just prior to the next set of vaccines or recommend that you give him acetaminophen as needed during the 24 hours after immunization.

 Although newborns may run a fever after receiving immunizations, check in with your pediatrician because any fever in a baby younger than 3 months should be evaluated. For older infants and toddlers, if fever persists for more than 24 hours or if the temperature is above 102°F (39°C), call your pediatrician. Very rare immunization side effects that warrant your pediatrician's attention include a rash all over the body, extensive swelling around the site of the shot or in the extremity used for the shot, persistent crying for more than a few hours, extreme lethargy, or seizure.

74. Can a high temperature cause brain damage?

Developing brain damage from fevers is an urban legend. Typical childhood fevers that are caused by infection do not cause brain damage. It takes an extremely high body temperature, such as over 108°F (42.2°C), to even potentially cause brain damage. This can occur with high environmental temperatures, such as those found in an enclosed car on a hot day, not typically from a common illness such as a cold or an ear infection.

75. My child had a seizure while sick with a fever. We took her to the emergency department. After examining her, the doctor told us it was a febrile seizure. What does this mean?

A febrile seizure is a type of seizure that occurs as the body temperature is quickly rising. During a seizure, your child may appear dazed, roll her eyes, stiffen, twitch, and/or shake (either the entire body or part of the body). Febrile seizures occur in fewer than 5% of children aged 6 months to 5 years. Children are more at risk for febrile seizure when their body temperature rises extremely quickly. In fact, many parents don't even realize that their child has a fever until they get to their pediatrician's office or the emergency department for evaluation of the child's seizure and the temperature is checked.

Although terrifying for parents to watch, febrile seizures are rarely dangerous and usually last less than 1 minute, but may occur for up to 15 minutes. They will not cause brain damage and will not affect future intelligence or behavior. Having a febrile seizure does not necessarily mean that your child is going to develop a seizure disorder. About 1 in 3 kids who have had a febrile seizure are at risk for having more seizures, especially if there is a family history of seizures or if the first seizure occurred at less than 1 year of age. Unfortunately, giving fever-reducing medicine like acetaminophen or ibuprofen when your child is sick does not seem to decrease the risk of having more febrile seizures. If your child has had a febrile seizure, ask your pediatrician for more information. And rest assured that nearly all kids outgrow the tendency to have febrile seizures.

 Although it may be stating the obvious, call your pediatrician the first time your child has a seizure, so your child can be thoroughly evaluated. If your child has a known history of febrile seizures, discuss how to manage future fevers or seizures with your pediatrician, including the need to call him or her if a seizure is different from previous episodes.

CHAPTER 8

Coughs, Colds, and More

Many children spend a good portion of their toddlerhood continuously coughing, with mucus running out of their nose. They seem to get better, they return to child care or preschool or attend a birthday party, and a few days later they are home with some new illness. Luckily, with immunizations protecting our little ones from many potentially serious and life-threatening infections, most of what they easily pick up these days will go away on its own (although it may first infect you and everyone else in your house).

It's never fun when one of your kids is sick (believe me, I know), especially because they always seem to be ill during an important work meeting or before a big family trip or event. So when can you wait to call your pediatrician? When should you call? And when do you need to seek medical attention right away? Here are the most common questions parents and caregivers ask about colds, coughs, and other similar illnesses.

Suddenly Sick

76. How do I know if my baby is sick?

Your baby can't tell you that he's not feeling well, but he will show you by changing his normal behavior. Sometimes the changes are subtle, and sometimes they're more obvious, but changes from your baby's normal behavior and routine will be your tip-off that something may not be right. He may drink less, cry more, sleep more or less, breathe faster, have a fever, or just not "look right." Babies, especially those younger than 28 days, are more susceptible to serious infections that can progress rapidly, so it is important to call your doctor right away if you notice anything unusual. Trust your instincts. You know your baby's behaviors better than anyone else, so let your pediatrician know if something doesn't seem right.

Call your pediatrician immediately if your newborn or young infant has a temperature of 100.4°F (38°C) or higher (see chapter 7, Fever, for more information and instructions on how to take your baby's temperature). Other reasons to call your doctor include the following:

☐ Excessive fussiness
☐ Continuous or high-pitched crying
☐ Poor feeding
☐ Extreme sleepiness (difficult to wake up to feed)
☐ Rapid breathing
☐ Decreased number of wet diapers

☐ Vomiting

☐ Sweating while feeding

☐ Any blueness of the skin, especially around the mouth

77. Why does it seem like my child is always sick? Could there be something wrong with her immune system?

Healthy kids (with normal immune systems) can catch about 10 infections a year, especially if they are in child care or preschool. During most summers (COVID-19 pandemic summers are an exception), they tend to be mostly well, but it's common for them to bring home a new illness every 2 or 3 weeks during the winter. With symptoms often lasting 1 to 2 weeks, sometimes it seems like they are always sick! Most of the usual suspects (coughs and colds) are caused by viruses and will clear up on their own. Children pick up colds from their friends or classmates—these viruses can survive on surfaces for hours and spread easily from person to person.

Often, children are contagious before they become symptomatic. So even if no one appears to be sick, there may still be some sharing of germs that can cause illness. If your child seems to follow this pattern of frequent illnesses, although it's a nuisance, it is unlikely that anything is wrong with her immune system. Children who have problems with their immune system usually have recurrent unusual infections (not regular colds and coughs), such as serious pneumonias, severe sinus infections, skin abscesses, or meningitis (an infection around the brain and spinal cord), that often require hospitalization and intravenous antibiotics.

If your infant or toddler has been hospitalized several times with serious infections that require antibiotics, talk to your pediatrician to find out if any special testing is needed.

Dr. Tanya's Tip
Keeping Kids Germ Free

☐ Wash hands after playing, after touching pets, when entering the house, before eating, after using the bathroom, and after sneezing, coughing, or blowing their nose.

☐ Carry hand sanitizer (also available with lotion) or wipes for times when soap and water aren't available. Rub hand sanitizer over the entire surface of the hands and wrists for at least 15 seconds and let them air dry.

☐ Remind children to cover coughs with the inside of their elbows (not their hands) and to wash their hands after wiping a runny nose.

☐ Wipe down commonly shared surfaces in your home (door handles, countertops, phones, and electronics) with a household cleaner that kills viruses.

78. My child has a cold. Can I give him over-the-counter cold medicine?

Over-the-counter cough and cold medications aren't generally recommended for babies and toddlers. They have not been proven to help treat colds, and there may be some unpleasant or potentially harmful side effects associated with them. Home remedies, herbal remedies, and supplements may also contain potentially dangerous ingredients, so always check with your pediatrician before giving anything to a young child.

If the cold is bothering your child, your best option is to try to clean out that stuffy nose so he can breathe and drink more easily. Place a drop or two of nasal saline in each nostril to loosen the mucus and help it drain. If the mucus is interfering with sleep or feeding, try gentle suctioning with a bulb or a nasal-oral aspirator (don't worry, there is a valve to keep the mucus from entering your mouth as you suck). He won't like it, but if you can get the gunk out, he'll feel better. Using a cool-mist humidifier or vaporizer at night may also help. The steam from a warm shower can also be helpful. For more tips on relieving nasal congestion and suctioning your little one's nose, refer to question 12 on page 23.

As always, when your child is sick, make sure he drinks plenty of fluids.

Call your pediatrician or make an appointment for your child if the following applies:

Your newborn or young infant (younger than 3 months) has cold symptoms that are interfering with eating or sleeping or has trouble breathing or a fever.

Your child is an infant older than 3 months and has a fever that persists for more than 3 to 4 days, cold symptoms that last longer than 5 to 7 days without improvement, or breathing that becomes very fast or seems labored.

It's often okay if cold symptoms (such as cough and runny nose) linger for more than a week in toddlers. Call if symptoms seem to be worsening after 5 to 7 days, if nasal discharge or congestion doesn't improve after 10 days, if the cold is keeping your toddler up at night, or if your toddler develops a new symptom such as a fever. In addition, your toddler should be evaluated for any fever that persists for more than 3 days or if a new fever appears after several days of having a cold.

Eyes and Ears and Mouth and Nose

79. My child woke up with red eyes and a green eye discharge. Is this pinkeye? Does she need eye drops? When can she return to preschool?

Pinkeye (conjunctivitis) is similar to a cold, but in the eye. It is very contagious and easily spreads from child to child because they often touch their eyes with contaminated hands. It can be caused by a virus, which will get better on its own, or a bacterium that needs to be treated with antibiotic eye medication. A good rule of thumb is that antibiotic eye medication may be needed if there is yellow or green discharge, especially if the eyelids are stuck shut on waking or if the discharge reappears within minutes of wiping. If the eyes are just red without any discharge or with clear discharge, you may be able to wait. It should clear up on its own within a few days. If your child also has a cold or fever, is uncomfortable, or isn't acting well, see your pediatrician because an ear or a sinus infection can sometimes accompany the eye infection.

 Call your pediatrician and describe your child's specific symptoms to see if your child needs an appointment or a prescription.

80. My baby has a cold and is tugging on his ears. Could he have an ear infection? Does he need an antibiotic?

In general, ear tugging is not a reliable indicator of an ear infection. However, if your baby has had a cold for several days and now has a fever, is fussy, is waking up at night, or is eating and drinking less in addition to the ear tugging, it's a good idea to have his ears checked. Even if he has had an ear infection before or was in the doctor's office yesterday for a cold, his ears need to be checked again. Ears can become infected overnight, so the findings of an ear examination can change in 1 day. Examining the ears is important because it helps doctors determine if an antibiotic is needed and, if so, which antibiotic to use. Not all ear infections require an antibiotic. Some are caused by a virus and will go away on their own. Depending on your child's age, other symptoms (eg, fever, pain), and how the ears look at the examination, your pediatrician will decide whether an antibiotic is needed (for a bacterial ear infection) or if a wait-and-see approach can be taken. With the wait-and-see approach, you may be instructed to call your pediatrician or start treatment if fever, pain, or other symptoms appear or if current symptoms worsen. Your pediatrician may advise you to bring your child back for an ear recheck a few days later or after any treatment is complete to determine if the infection is truly gone and if any fluid remains.

It is true that some children are just more prone to ear infections than others. However, certain factors can increase your child's risk, such as going to bed with a bottle, attending child care, and being exposed to secondhand smoke. How can you decrease your child's risk of developing ear infections? If possible, avoid these risk factors in the following ways:

☐ Do not put your child to bed with a bottle.
☐ Do not allow your child to be exposed to secondhand smoke.

☐ Reduce or eliminate pacifier use after 6 months of age (this has been shown to reduce recurrent ear infections).

☐ Vaccinate your child against pneumococcus and influenza. In addition to preventing these diseases, these vaccinations help children develop fewer ear infections during respiratory illness season, which is when most ear infections occur.

☐ Breastfeed your infant for at least the first 6 months if possible to help prevent ear infections— one more reason to breastfeed your little one!

81. My child is prone to ear infections. Does she need ear tubes?

Possibly. Ear tubes (pressure equalization tubes, sometimes called *myringotomy tubes* or *tympanostomy tubes*) may significantly reduce the number of ear infections a child develops and prevent hearing loss. It's amazing how they can change your child's (and your) life. Your pediatrician may recommend that your child see a specialist about having ear tubes placed if she has recurrent infections, persistent infection that can't be cleared with antibiotic use, persistent fluid behind the eardrum, complications from infections, or hearing or speech delay.

During this simple and common surgery, small tubes (the tubes are tiny and short—they're more like grommets) are placed in the eardrums to allow air to get behind the eardrum and fluid to drain as needed. They typically fall out with time, and the eardrum heals on its own.

> ## Middle-Ear Versus Outer-Ear Infection
>
> **Middle-Ear Infection: Otitis Media**
>
> This occurs when fluid becomes infected behind the eardrum. This type of infection is more likely to occur when your child has a cold.
>
> **Outer-Ear Infection: Otitis Externa (Swimmer's Ear)**
>
> This occurs when the skin lining the ear canal becomes infected. It is usually caused by water getting trapped or by trauma (such as from a cotton swab); bacteria then grow. Outer-ear infections are very painful, especially when you touch or tug on the ear. Treatment involves the use of antibiotic ear drops.

82. My child has an ear infection. When can he take a bath or go swimming?

That depends on the type of ear infection your child has: See the text box about middle-ear infection versus outer-ear infection. Most ear infections that young children get are middle-ear infections, which means the infection is behind the eardrum. In this case, bathing your child, getting water in his ear, or swimming shouldn't make the ear infection worse or prevent it from getting better. If your child also has discharge leaking from the ear or if your pediatrician said the eardrum was perforated or punctured, then she may recommend *(a)* not swimming, *(b)* not letting your child dip his head underwater, *(c)* not pouring water over his head while bathing, or *(d)* not doing anything where water might get into the ear canal. If your child has an external or outer-ear infection, otherwise known as *swimmer's ear,* your doctor may recommend avoiding swimming or getting water in his ears for a few days while it heals. Eventually you might want to consider ear plugs for swimming. A bath is fine, as long as your child doesn't submerge his head underwater.

If your child seems uncomfortable swimming or if water that gets in the ear during a bath seems to cause pain, then hold off and let your pediatrician take a look.

83. My child has a fever and is refusing to drink. I think his throat or mouth is hurting. What should I do?

Many infections can cause your little one's mouth or throat to hurt. For children younger than 3 years, most infections are viral and will improve on their own in about a week. The most important thing to do is keep him well-hydrated, so let him drink anything that he likes. Some children need a little encouragement, but most can be coaxed to take small sips with a straw. Popsicles work well too! Your pediatrician may also recommend giving him acetaminophen or ibuprofen for the pain.

Here's a rundown on the most common sore throat or mouth illnesses.

☐ **Hand, foot, and mouth disease:** In addition to having a fever for a few days with painful sores in the mouth, your child often will develop a blister-like rash on the hands, feet, and sometimes the diaper area. The rash may also be tender, especially on the bottom of the feet, so your child may not want to walk. Fortunately, the discomfort will soon pass, and nothing needs to be applied to the rash. All symptoms are caused by a coxsackievirus infection and will improve on their own. Your pediatrician may advise you to try giving your child acetaminophen or ibuprofen for the discomfort.

☐ **Sore throat and pink eyes:** Again, these symptoms are usually caused by a virus, typically adenovirus, to be exact. The back of the throat can look very red and may even have pus on it. It is not strep throat (which is caused by a bacterial infection) and does not require antibiotics to heal. The virus also causes the white part of the eyes to look pink, sometimes with a sticky discharge. These pink eyes need no treatment and will get better on their own. This virus can also cause ear infections and an upset stomach.

☐ **Major mouth ulcers:** Although several viruses can cause a few white ulcers (sores) in the mouth or throat, if your child's mouth and tongue are covered with them and he is in lots of pain, he may have a common childhood herpes simplex virus infection (different from genital herpes). In some cases, an antiviral medication or a pain reliever may be prescribed. It is essential that you encourage your child to drink liquids. Despite everyone's best efforts, some children are in so much discomfort that they will completely refuse to drink anything. In such cases, it may be necessary to hospitalize your child so he may receive intravenous fluids and pain medications.

☐ **Strep throat:** Strep throat is not common in children younger than 3 years unless a close family member has it and gives it to your child. Strep throat symptoms are a fever and a sore throat *without* cold symptoms (runny nose and cough). There may also be stomach pain, headache, vomiting, or a rash. Strep throat with a rash is called *scarlet fever*. It sounds scary, but it is treated with the same antibiotics used for regular strep throat. Reassure your child's grandparents that because we now have antibiotics to treat the infection, scarlet fever is no longer as dangerous as it was years ago!

 As always, call or see your pediatrician if your newborn or young infant has a fever, is drinking less, refuses 2 or more feedings in a row, or looks sick.

For children older than 3 months, call or see your pediatrician if the fever lasts more than 3 days, if your child isn't drinking well, or if he looks really sick.

84. My child has green nasal discharge. Does she need an antibiotic?

Despite what your mother may have told you, green mucus does not always mean antibiotics are needed. Plenty of viruses (common colds) cause green mucus that goes away on its own. If your child has a runny nose with clear mucus for more than a week or two and then it turns yellow or green, or if she suddenly develops a fever after not having one for the first few days of her illness, or if it seems like she is in pain (eg, she is fussy or irritable), she should be examined because she may have developed a sinus infection or an ear infection. Please don't ask for an antibiotic to be prescribed over the phone. Your child should always be examined first to know exactly what is going on and what needs to be treated.

Coughing and Wheezing

85. My child wheezes and coughs when he gets a cold. Does this mean he has asthma?

Possibly. Colds (also called *upper respiratory tract infections*) are the most common cause of wheezing in infants and toddlers. Their small airways easily get inflamed and narrow when triggered by an infection. Sometimes, a viral infection that causes wheezing in an infant or a young toddler may be called *bronchiolitis* (discussed more in the next section). Most physicians will call it *asthma* after a few wheezing episodes or if the wheezing recurs over a period of several months or years. If your child has frequent or reoccurring wheezing, asthma medications may be needed to help your child breathe more easily and prevent future episodes of wheezing. A bronchodilator (such as albuterol or levalbuterol) is often given via a nebulizer or an inhaler with spacer to help open the airways and make it easier for your child to breathe during an episode.

If your child's wheezing is recurring or only improving a little with a bronchodilator, oral steroids may be needed for a few days to decrease the inflammation and mucus in your child's lungs. For children who have frequent or severe episodes, daily medications (inhaled or oral) may be prescribed to protect the airways, decrease inflammation at baseline, and prevent wheezing year-round or at least during the winter months, when colds are more prevalent. As your child grows, the airways grow, and this problem may go away. If you have a family history of asthma, allergies, or eczema, there is a chance that your child's symptoms will persist and he will officially receive a diagnosis of asthma.

 Let your pediatrician know if you think your child may be wheezing. The doctor will listen to your child's lungs and prescribe appropriate treatment.

86. What is RSV? Is my child at risk?

RSV stands for *respiratory syncytial virus.* In older
children and adults, it causes a cold with a really
runny, goopy nose—the one you get almost every
winter. In young children, the infection can cause
minor cold symptoms to serious lung problems—
usually depending on the child's age and medical
history (such as premature birth, heart disease,
or lung disease). RSV is most common during the
winter.

In newborns and infants, RSV infection of the lungs
can be one of many common causes of bronchiolitis,
an inflammation and infection of the tiny airways of
the lungs caused by any number of viral infections. It
can cause wheezing and serious difficulty breathing,
especially in babies who were born early (prematurely)
and have problems with their immune systems or
those who have heart or lung disease. For these high-
risk babies, there is a shot available called *palivizumab*
(Synagis) to help protect them from catching RSV. It
is given once a month, usually from October through
April, when RSV is most prevalent. Ask your pediatrician if your infant qualifies.

When it comes to toddlers and preschoolers with
RSV, most will have a runny, goopy nose. Some may
develop bronchiolitis (as discussed for newborns and
infants) but can usually be cared for at home after being
examined by the pediatrician. Because RSV is a virus,
as long as there is no associated trouble breathing,

the illness will improve on its own. (See the next question for tips on managing RSV infection and bronchiolitis.) RSV is extremely contagious, so it is a good idea to keep your toddler away from newborns and help her frequently wash her hands.

87. What is the treatment for bronchiolitis if my child does get it?

There is no medication to treat bronchiolitis or RSV. Only symptomatic care, such as gentle suctioning of the mucus from the nose, has been shown to help. Other important steps include treating a fever if it is making your child uncomfortable (see chapter 7, Fever, for recommendations), making sure that your child is drinking well, and allowing your child to rest.

In the past, medications used to treat wheezing caused by asthma were given to try to treat wheezing caused by bronchiolitis; however, these medications have been shown to be of limited effectiveness and are not routinely recommended for treatment of wheezing from bronchiolitis.

Some infants and children have severe responses to viral infections and develop difficulty breathing (manifested as fast, shallow breathing; use of chest and neck muscles to breathe; and difficulty eating and drinking). Monitoring these children in the hospital is usually recommended, where they can be supported with extra oxygen, breathing treatments, or fluids as needed.

Call your pediatrician right away if any of the following is true:

☐ Your newborn or infant has a cold and is breathing fast (more than 60 times a minute).

☐ You hear wheezing or notice retractions, where the skin is being sucked in above or below the ribs with each breath.

☐ Your child is having trouble eating, drinking, or sleeping.

☐ Your child is making 3 or fewer wet diapers in 24 hours.

If your toddler has any wheezing or trouble breathing, call your pediatrician. In addition, if your toddler is so sick that she cannot drink enough to have normal urine output (at least 4 wet diapers in 24 hours), then call your pediatrician to evaluate your child for possible dehydration.

88. My child has a bad cough. Should I bring him to the doctor? How do I know if he has pneumonia?

Many coughs are caused by postnasal drip from a cold rather than an actual lung infection, such as pneumonia. So how do you know the difference? In general, if your child has a runny nose and is acting well between bouts of coughing, you may be able to just keep an eye on him at home. Although a cough can sometimes linger for a few weeks, it shouldn't be getting any worse after 4 or 5 days. If your child starts to breathe fast, if the cough isn't beginning to improve after a week or is worsening, or if a new fever appears, be sure to have your doctor examine your child because sometimes serious infections can develop, such as pneumonia. In such cases, antibiotics may be needed to treat the infection.

 Call your doctor right away if there are any signs of troubled breathing, such as wheezing, grunting, skin being sucked in above or below the ribs when your child is breathing (retractions), stomach moving in and out with each breath, or chest pain. In addition, if your child's cough is keeping him up all night or if he has a high fever, call for an appointment.

89. My child woke up in the middle of the night with a horrible, barking cough—like a seal. What is it?

In general, a "seal bark" indicates croup. Croup is a viral infection (often caused by parainfluenza virus) that causes swelling of the upper airway, voice box, and windpipe (not the lungs). It produces a distinctive barky, seal-like cough and a hoarse voice. Older kids and adults usually develop only a loud cough and a hoarse voice or just cold symptoms. Because it's a virus, antibiotics won't help.

In newborns, infants, and toddlers, the inflammation can sometimes be severe enough to produce stridor—a loud, harsh, high-pitched sound heard when your child breathes in that may be associated with trouble breathing. This can occur at rest when your child is playing or feeding or when he is agitated or fussy. The second or third night of coughing tends to be the worst. Even though your child might seem fine during the day, it's important to talk to your pediatrician to find out if treatment is needed.

To help decrease stridor, spend 20 minutes with your child outside in the cool night air or in a steam-filled bathroom. Running a humidifier or vaporizer in her bedroom at night may also help.

 If the stridor isn't improving or if it worsens, if your child has a high fever or trouble breathing, or if your child can't swallow well or is drooling, call your pediatrician, go to the emergency department, or call 911. Your child may need a steroid medication or a special inhaled treatment to decrease the inflammation in the airway and make it easier to breathe.

90. What can I do at home to help my child's cough?

I know it's hard to hear your child cough, especially in the middle of the night. If your child isn't bothered by the cough, isn't having trouble breathing, is acting well, and is sleeping well at night (despite coughing), try not to let it bother you, and give it some time to get better on its own.

Coughing happens because something (either a virus or something in the environment) is irritating the airway. As the irritant goes away, the cough does, too. If the symptoms are bothersome or uncomfortable for your child or if they keep him awake at night, giving him something to ease the cough may help.

In general, cough medicines (even those marketed for kids!) should not be given to infants, toddlers, and young kids since they have not been shown to reduce cough or cold symptoms; they have many unpleasant side effects; and they can lead to severe problems if taken too often. Even medicines that are labeled "natural" may not be helpful for cough and may contain compounds that are dangerous or harmful for young children.

There are some safe options for helping your child feel better. Supportive care (as described previously in the section on RSV), including use of nasal saline, suctioning of nasal mucus, good fluid intake, and rest, can be helpful. Placing saline drops in your child's nose can help loosen up mucus and help with cough, as can breathing in warm steam from the shower. If the air in your house is dry, using a humidifier can also help to soothe irritated airways and decrease coughing (just remember to clean the humidifier regularly to prevent mold growth in the water). For older infants and toddlers, 1 to 3 teaspoons of warm fluids (water, juice, herbal tea, or other clear liquid) can be given by mouth every 6 hours or so to soothe coughing.

Honey can also be helpful for children *older than 12 months*. Giving your child ½ to 1 teaspoon of honey as needed has been shown to decrease night-time coughing and help children sleep better at night. In a study about cough treatments for children, honey worked better than any store-bought cough medicine tested—and it tastes great!

Important Note About Honey

Do not give honey to your newborn or infant if she is younger than 12 months old. Infants younger than 12 months who eat honey can develop infant botulism, a disease that causes weakness and paralysis and is sometimes bad enough to necessitate breathing tubes and feeding tubes to support a child through the illness.

Is Nighttime Cough Keeping You Up?

A nighttime cough without a fever or other symptoms may not be an infection. A cough, especially at night, is a common hallmark of asthma. Coughing can also indicate drainage from the nose or sinuses into the throat while lying down, which could be caused by allergies or an infection (cold or sinus). In other cases, it can also be a sign of reflux (see question 40). Usually, your pediatrician can obtain a thorough history and perform an examination to determine the cause of the cough and provide treatment as needed.

CHAPTER 9

Vaccines

As a mom, I know it can be hard to expose your little one to pokes and pain. And there are a lot of opinions regarding vaccines. Whether you're reading this before your little one arrives or even afterward, you may be thinking about your grandfather who survived polio but walked with a cane or the amusement park measles outbreak that occurred a few years ago, or you may be thinking, "But my neighbor's cousin's daughter said . . ." So here are the most common questions I hear from new parents about vaccines.

91. What vaccines should I get as a new parent/ grandparent/caregiver?

It's important that everyone who cares for a new baby is protected against whooping cough (also known as pertussis) and the flu (influenza), as both of these illnesses can cause serious infections, trouble breathing, and even death in young babies. Both vaccines are safe to get during pregnancy, for the protection of both mom and baby. Although the influenza vaccine can be given at any time during pregnancy (ideally right at the beginning of flu season), the pertussis vaccine should be given in the last trimester of pregnancy to pass antibodies from mom to baby just before birth.

Many adults are no longer protected against whooping cough because immunity to pertussis (whether you were previously vaccinated or actually had whooping cough) wears off with time. Often, infected adults have a lingering cough that they don't realize is whooping cough until a baby catches it, at which point the baby can get very sick and even stop breathing. Influenza is similar in that the virus changes enough from year to year that your body cannot recognize and protect against it; thus, your previous protection against the influenza virus does not carry forward (hence the need for a new flu shot every year!). Infants who catch influenza can become very sick, sometimes necessitating admission to the intensive care unit or placement of a breathing tube to be able to make it through the illness.

Infants can't receive their own first pertussis vaccine until 2 months of age and are not eligible for the flu vaccine until 6 months of age, so the best way to protect your baby is to protect yourself. If you, your family members, or your child's caregivers are missing any vaccines from childhood, discussing this with your doctor during pregnancy or even before pregnancy is good so that everyone can catch up on missed vaccines and provide the best protection possible for your baby. If your baby has already arrived, don't worry—you and your family members can catch up on your vaccines

now, as well. Don't take chances; if you vaccinate
everyone in your home, you form a protective shield
around your newborn and decrease the risk that your
baby will catch these very serious illnesses.

92. Why should I vaccinate my child?

Thanks to vaccines, many diseases that once caused
death and disability in children are now rare in the
United States. However, although these diseases may
be rare here, they aren't gone. Many of these infections remain common in other countries and are thus
only a plane ride away, just waiting to make a come-
back, which will happen if people stop vaccinating. I
have seen previously healthy children get seriously
ill, become permanently disabled, and even die of
diseases, such as meningitis, chickenpox, and whooping cough, that could have been prevented by getting
vaccinated. By vaccinating your child, you are protecting not only your own child but also others who are
at increased risk, such as newborns, friends who are
undergoing chemotherapy, and elderly grandparents.

93. Why are there so many vaccines? When I was
a child, there were only a few. Are kids today
getting too many vaccines?

Great question. We are indeed protecting against more
diseases today—children now receive vaccines to protect against 14 diseases. These are diseases that I don't
want my own children or my patients to experience.

However, I find that parents are surprised to learn that all the vaccines that kids get today, combined, are actually less potent than *one* vaccine I got as a child (and I'm older than you!). It's true—all of these vaccines together are less of an immunologic challenge to the body than the few vaccines I got when I was young, or the several you received when you were young. That's because vaccines have been purified over the years, thanks to vaccine science. So today, kids receive about 150 proteins with all vaccines, in total, to stimulate their immune system. Just one vaccine when I was a child contained more than that. And this is a tiny drop in the bucket when compared to what kids' immune systems are exposed to on a daily basis, from just being out and about in the environment.

94. Are there any side effects from vaccines?

Overall, vaccines are very safe, but they may have minor side effects. Your child may experience soreness at the injection site, have a mild fever, be slightly cranky, or even sleep a little longer than usual (enjoy this one!) the day or two after some vaccines are given. Your pediatrician may recommend giving an appropriate dose of acetaminophen or, if your baby is older than 6 months, ibuprofen, as needed later that day for any pain or fussiness. Another common side effect from any shot is a pea-sized lump under the skin at the injection site. This is not dangerous and will resolve over the next few weeks.

The risk of developing a serious side effect from a vaccine is very small when compared with the risk of serious illness caused by catching the disease that the vaccine protects against. Countless medical studies support the safety of vaccines and show that vaccines do *not* cause autism or any other childhood disease. All vaccines recommended for use in children must undergo thorough investigation and licensing by the US Food and Drug Administration (FDA); each batch of vaccines is tested for safety and effectiveness before it is shipped out for use, and the FDA performs periodic inspections of the facilities that manufacture vaccines.

 Call your pediatrician if your child experiences any of the following symptoms after receiving vaccines: fever for more than 24 hours or temperature above 103°F (39.4°C), inconsolable crying for more than 3 hours, extreme lethargy, rash all over the body, seizure, or extensive swelling around the shot or in the extremity in which the shot was given.

95. Do vaccines cause autism?

To wrap up the autism debate, there is absolutely *no* link between vaccines and autism. The original article that claimed there was a connection between vaccines and autism was based on observations in only 12 children, and—what's worse—further investigations have shown that much data was completely made up! After it was discovered that the data in that article could not be reproduced in repeat studies, the research team was investigated, the article was retracted, and the doctor (who had performed unnecessary procedures on the children he was studying) was convicted of unethical behavior and barred from practicing medicine. Since then, numerous legitimate studies have shown no link between vaccines and autism, in both the United States and abroad.

96. Are there still ingredients, such as thimerosal and aluminum, in vaccines?

Thimerosal is a mercury-based organic compound that has been used to prevent microbes like bacteria and viruses from contaminating vaccines. Thimerosal has been studied in depth, and it is not stored anywhere in the human body or toxic to the body; it is also removed from the vaccine at the end of the manufacturing process, leaving only a tiny amount behind. However, because of concerns about even low-level exposure to compounds that contain mercury, the FDA recommended removing thimerosal from vaccines as a precautionary measure.

Today, thimerosal is no longer used in most vaccines, and it was removed from all childhood vaccines in 2001; therefore, none of the vaccines that your little one will receive should contain this preservative.

Aluminum salts help the body create a better immune response to vaccines and ultimately minimize the doses of shots babies need to be protected.

Aluminum is a naturally occurring substance from the earth's crust and is commonly found in the environment. We actually have varying amounts of aluminum in our bodies just from breathing air, drinking water, and eating foods like vegetables, which naturally contain aluminum. In fact, our babies are exposed to more aluminum in just 1 year of drinking breast milk than in all of the vaccines they are given in the first year!

97. Can we split, space out, or delay my baby's shots?

The current vaccination schedule in the United States has been fully researched and designed to provide the best immunity for your baby. We wouldn't be recommending these vaccines otherwise! If you delay your baby's shots, there won't be the right amount of protection at the exact times needed to keep your baby safe and healthy. Plus, splitting up shots means coming back and giving your baby another visit to cry at. There's no harm in receiving multiple vaccines at one visit! In fact, some work better when given together. Your baby will not remember a thing about getting his shots, and he will be happy and healthy because you made the right choice in getting him vaccinated on time.

98. My baby has a runny nose. Can she still get her shots?

Usually, the answer is yes! We do recommend that all babies get their shots on time unless they are seriously ill. In that case, your baby would need to be further evaluated by your pediatrician. Normal congestion in a baby is not a concern when it's time for vaccines. Even when your baby is older and starts picking up the occasional cold, as long as she doesn't have a high fever (a low-grade fever is okay, as long as your child looks well), is breathing comfortably, and isn't acting sick, it's okay for her to get her shots.

 Whether your newborn has recently received vaccines or not, if a newborn has a fever, or if a baby of any age is having trouble breathing, is not feeding well, or is acting sick, see your pediatrician immediately to get her checked out.

99. What about the yearly flu shot? Is it really necessary? Is there a possibility that my child could get sick from it?

The annual influenza vaccine is recommended for everyone 6 months of age and older not only as the best way to protect against the flu but also as a way to reduce the risk of flu-related infections, hospitalizations, and deaths. Flu shots can be given to anyone 6 months and older.

You can help protect babies younger than 6 months from the flu by making sure that everyone around them gets a flu vaccine, including siblings, parents, grandparents, caregivers, and anyone else who will be

around your little one. If your child is younger than 9
months and this is the first year he is getting a flu vaccine, 2 doses will be needed, 1 month apart, as
the first dose helps prime the immune system and the
second helps the body develop antibodies.

And no, you can't catch the flu from the flu shot.
Because the flu shot does not contain any live virus,
it cannot infect you. Lots of viruses are floating
around your home, school, and doctor's office in
the winter when we give the flu vaccine, though, so
people often catch something else around the same
time they get their shot and think that the shot made
them sick.

100. Who should get the COVID vaccine?

Everyone 6 months and older is eligible for a
vaccine to protect against COVID-19 infection. This
vaccine not only decreases the chance of catching
COVID, but it also decreases the chance of serious
complications from COVID infection. If everyone in
your household who is eligible for the COVID vaccine
gets it, this will also help protect anyone who is at
high risk for serious illness, disease, hospitalization,
and death from COVID-19. If you are pregnant or
breastfeeding, the COVID-19 vaccine is safe and
recommended, as antibodies that you make will help
protect you and also pass through and help protect
your baby. Vaccines are our best hope for ending
the pandemic.

Immunizations (aka Vaccines or Shots)

The table on the following 2 pages is a list of the vaccines recommended in the first 3 years after birth and why each one is important. Your pediatrician may have a slightly different immunization schedule, and some vaccines may be available in combination shots (which means fewer pokes for your little one!).

For more information on vaccines, speak with your pediatrician and visit the American Academy of Pediatrics website for parents (www.healthychildren.org) and the Centers for Disease Control and Prevention website (www.cdc.gov).

2022 Recommended Immunizations for Children from Birth Through 6 Years Old

	Birth	1 month	2 months	4 months	6 months	12 months	15 months	18 months	19-23 months	2-3 years	4-6 years
	HepB	HepB			HepB						
			RV	RV	RV						
			DTaP	DTaP	DTaP		DTaP				DTaP
			Hib	Hib	Hib	Hib					
			PCV13	PCV13	PCV13	PCV13					
			IPV	IPV	IPV						IPV
					Influenza (Yearly)*						
						MMR					MMR
						Varicella					Varicella
							HepA§				

Is your family growing? To protect your new baby against whooping cough, get a Tdap vaccine. The recommended time is the 27th through 36th week of pregnancy. Talk to your doctor for more details.

Shaded boxes indicate the vaccine can be given during shown age range.

NOTE:
If your child misses a shot, you don't need to start over. Just go back to your child's doctor for the next shot. Talk with your child's doctor if you have questions about vaccines.

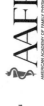

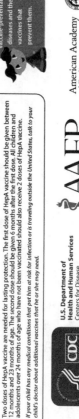

See back page for more information on vaccine-preventable diseases and the vaccines that prevent them.

COVID-19 VACCINATION IS RECOMMENDED FOR AGES 5 YEARS AND OLDER.

FOOTNOTES:

* Two doses given at least four weeks apart are recommended for children age 6 months through 8 years of age who are getting an influenza (flu) vaccine for the first time and for some other children in this age group.

§ Two doses of HepA vaccine are needed for lasting protection. The first dose of HepA vaccine should be given between 12 months and 23 months of age. The second dose should be given 6 months after the first dose. All children and adolescents over 24 months of age who have not been vaccinated should also receive 2 doses of HepA vaccine.

If your child has any medical conditions that put him at risk for infection or is traveling outside the United States, talk to your child's doctor about additional vaccines that he or she may need.

For more information, call toll-free
1-800-CDC-INFO (1-800-232-4636)
or visit
www.cdc.gov/vaccines/parents

U.S. Department of Health and Human Services
Centers for Disease Control and Prevention

American Academy of Pediatrics
DEDICATED TO THE HEALTH OF ALL CHILDREN™

AAFP
AMERICAN ACADEMY OF FAMILY PHYSICIANS

Vaccine-Preventable Diseases and the Vaccines that Prevent Them

Disease	Vaccine	Disease spread by	Disease symptoms	Disease complications
Chickenpox	Varicella vaccine protects against chickenpox.	Air, direct contact	Rash, tiredness, headache, fever	Infected blisters, bleeding disorders, encephalitis (brain swelling), pneumonia (infection in the lungs), death
Diphtheria	DTaP* vaccine protects against diphtheria.	Air, direct contact	Sore throat, mild fever, weakness, swollen glands in neck	Swelling of the heart muscle, heart failure, coma, paralysis, death
Hib	Hib vaccine protects against Haemophilus influenzae type b.	Air, direct contact	May be no symptoms unless bacteria enter the blood	Meningitis (infection of the covering around the brain and spinal cord), intellectual disability, epiglottitis (life-threatening infection that can block the windpipe and lead to serious breathing problems), pneumonia (infection in the lungs), death
Hepatitis A	HepA vaccine protects against hepatitis A.	Direct contact, contaminated food or water	May be no symptoms, fever, stomach pain, loss of appetite, fatigue, vomiting, jaundice (yellowing of skin and eyes), dark urine	Liver failure, arthralgia (joint pain), kidney, pancreatic and blood disorders, death
Hepatitis B	HepB vaccine protects against hepatitis B.	Contact with blood or body fluids	May be no symptoms, fever, headache, weakness, vomiting, jaundice (yellowing of skin and eyes), joint pain	Chronic liver infection, liver failure, liver cancer, death
Influenza (Flu)	Flu vaccine protects against influenza.	Air, direct contact	Fever, muscle pain, sore throat, cough, extreme fatigue	Pneumonia (infection in the lungs), bronchitis, sinus infections, ear infections, death
Measles	MMR** vaccine protects against measles.	Air, direct contact	Rash, fever, cough, runny nose, pink eye	Encephalitis (brain swelling), pneumonia (infection in the lungs), death
Mumps	MMR**vaccine protects against mumps.	Air, direct contact	Swollen salivary glands (under the jaw), fever, headache, tiredness, muscle pain	Meningitis (infection of the covering around the brain and spinal cord), encephalitis (brain swelling), inflammation of testicles or ovaries, deafness, death
Pertussis	DTaP* vaccine protects against pertussis (whooping cough).	Air, direct contact	Severe cough, runny nose, apnea (a pause in breathing in infants)	Pneumonia (infection in the lungs), death
Polio	IPV vaccine protects against polio.	Air, direct contact, through the mouth	May be no symptoms, sore throat, fever, nausea, headache	Paralysis, death
Pneumococcal	PCV13 vaccine protects against pneumococcus.	Air, direct contact	May be no symptoms, pneumonia (infection in the lungs)	Bacteremia (blood infection), meningitis (infection of the covering around the brain and spinal cord), death
Rotavirus	RV vaccine protects against rotavirus.	Through the mouth	Diarrhea, fever, vomiting	Severe diarrhea, dehydration, death
Rubella	MMR** vaccine protects against rubella.	Air, direct contact	Sometimes rash, fever, swollen lymph nodes	Very serious in pregnant women—can lead to miscarriage, stillbirth, premature delivery, birth defects
Tetanus	DTaP* vaccine protects against tetanus.	Exposure through cuts in skin	Stiffness in neck and abdominal muscles, difficulty swallowing, muscle spasms, fever	Broken bones, breathing difficulty, death

* DTaP combines protection against diphtheria, tetanus, and pertussis.
** MMR combines protection against measles, mumps, and rubella.

Last updated February 2022 - CS322257-A

CHAPTER 10

Skin

After soaking in amniotic fluid for 9 months (kind of like an extended spa vacation), you'd expect your newborn to have silky, soft, clear skin. While some do, more often than not, babies have dry, cracked skin that may develop an assortment of bumps and blemishes throughout the first year or so. Although many of these rashes are completely normal and resolve on their own, other skin conditions can pop up during the first few years. Some are a result of dry weather or irritating soaps. Many come hand in hand with a variety of viral illnesses picked up from playmates or siblings. And some rashes occur for no apparent reason at all.

Even though the red blotches may not bother the affected child, rashes in general can be bothersome for parents and caregivers. My general rule of thumb is that if the rash isn't bothering the child, it doesn't bother me. However, a trip to the pediatrician may be needed for evaluation and to obtain a note stating when it is safe to return to child care or preschool.

The following questions and answers help demystify some of the more common red or dry patches you may discover under your child's clothes. Often when it comes to a rash, a picture is worth a thousand words. So don't be surprised if you need to snap a photo or take a trip to your pediatrician's office to get to the bottom of the blotch. (If your child has a cut, scrape, or bite, see chapter 12, Ingestions, Injuries, and First Aid.)

Jaundice

101. My newborn is yellow. My mother says it is "jaundice." What does that mean? Should I be worried?

Your mom is right. The yellowish color of the skin is called *jaundice*, a common occurrence in newborns. The first hint of yellow typically appears on the face and then progresses down the body. In otherwise healthy infants, it is usually at its worst around day 4 or 5 and then begins to resolve, although the yellow color of the face and in the whites of the eyes (called *scleral icterus*) can linger for a week or two.

It may reassure you to know that most babies turn a bit yellow after birth; some are just more noticeable than others. It develops from a normal process that occurs in all babies involving the breakdown of red blood cells. The normal breakdown of red blood cells produces a substance called bilirubin. This process occurs in the liver and the bilirubin is excreted in the intestines (in your baby's poop!). Because this excretion process is very immature, some babies just can't keep up, and extra bilirubin lingers in the blood and then gets deposited in the skin, causing the yellow color.

Jaundice can be more pronounced in babies who were born early (4 weeks early or more to be exact) or have bruising from the birthing process (especially if they have a large head bruise, called a *cephalohematoma*). Babies are also at an increased risk of developing jaundice if they have a sibling who had significant jaundice as a newborn, if mom has blood type O+ and baby has a different blood type (called *ABO incompatibility*), or if they are of East Asian descent.

Although some degree of jaundice is normal in newborns, it can sometimes indicate a more serious problem, such as infection, liver disease, or blood disorders. That is why it is important to let your pediatrician know if your baby begins to look yellow. In addition to compiling a quick history and performing a physical examination, your pediatrician may need to perform a simple blood or skin test to help determine your baby's bilirubin level and enable her to advise on any necessary treatment.

The most common reason for jaundice is breastfeeding jaundice. This usually occurs in the first week when the baby is not taking in enough milk, either because mom's milk supply is not fully in or because the baby has yet to master the art of nursing. Your pediatrician may advise you to increase the frequency of your breastfeeding sessions or even give your baby temporary supplemental expressed breast milk or formula to make sure he receives enough liquid to poop adequately and clear out the bilirubin. If your baby is jaundiced, it is particularly important to not let him sleep past 3 hours without feeding. If you are having difficulty keeping your baby with jaundice awake, despite trying things like tickling his feet, getting him undressed, or changing his diaper, let your pediatrician know as soon as possible. It is important to note that many mothers have successfully breastfed their infants after giving them supplemental formula in the immediate newborn period. In addition, nursing near a window, with your baby in indirect sunlight, can help to break down bilirubin in the skin a little.

The take-home message is: The more your baby eats and poops, the more bilirubin will be cleared from the body, and the sooner the jaundice will resolve.

In contrast, jaundice that develops within the first 24 hours of birth or outside of the immediate newborn period (after the first 3–4 weeks) is not normal and should be evaluated by your pediatrician as soon as possible, because it could be a sign of rapid breakdown of red blood cells, infection, or liver disease. If you think your infant or toddler's skin has a yellow or orange hue, but the whites of her eyes are still white (no scleral icterus), you can relax, as chances are the skin is discolored from eating too many carotene-containing foods, such as carrots, sweet potatoes, and squash. In this case, you may notice that your child's palms, soles, and face (especially the tip of her nose) are a little more yellow than the rest of her body. There is no need to intervene, except maybe to back off a little on yellow and orange veggies in favor of green ones.

 Let your pediatrician know if your baby starts to look yellow, so the doctor can assess the situation and check the bilirubin level if needed. In some instances, newborns with high bilirubin levels may benefit from extra fluids or require treatment with special lights (called phototherapy) or a special light blanket in the hospital or at home.

However, if your infant or toddler has true jaundice (yellow skin and eyes), call your pediatrician as soon as possible.

Rashes

102. What are the best creams for diaper rash?

The diaper cream you choose will depend on the type of diaper rash your baby has. In the first week after birth, diaper rashes are often simply caused by irritation from wetness. Applying a cream that contains zinc oxide is generally best for creating a barrier between a baby's sensitive skin and irritants, but even a thin layer of petroleum jelly or nonpetroleum ointment can work well in preventing many common newborn rashes (not to mention helpful in making stool easier to wipe off!).

If, however, your baby has a rash that is bright reddish pink and raised or sometimes raw, often with little bumps surrounding it, chances are you're looking at a yeast infection. In such cases, you will need a special yeast cream (see question 103). Whenever your baby's diaper rash doesn't improve after a few days with the cream of your choice, or if you have questions about how to best treat a rash in the first place, be sure to call your pediatrician.

Dr. Tanya's Tip
Sensitive Baby Bottoms

Years ago, damp gauze pads were used in the hospital instead of wipes to clean a newborn's sensitive bottom. Now, it's fairly commonplace for hospitals to have samples of baby wipes that are gentle enough to use from day 1. Alcohol-free, unscented baby wipes made with only a few ingredients including water are fine. If your newborn develops irritation or a rash, dipping gauze pads, a very soft paper towel, or a soft baby washcloth (if you're okay with washing the washcloths afterward) in warm water works well for cleaning sensitive bottoms. This tip also comes in handy for older infants and toddlers with really impressive diaper rashes that tend to linger. Sometimes, laying off the wipes for a few days to a week, having some diaper-free time at home, and switching back to soft cloths or paper towels can help.

103. Why do babies get rashes from yeast, and how do I clear it up?

Yeast grows best in warm, moist places like your baby's diaper area! The typical yeast rash is hot pink or red, raised, and quite "angry" looking. Often, several small spots extend beyond the main area of the rash. A yeast rash is caused by a type of yeast called *Candida albicans*. While this infection of the skin is common in babies and causes its fair share of distress (for babies and their parents), it is fortunately not truly dangerous. Getting rid of a yeast infection requires a special antifungal cream. I find that using a combination antifungal and diaper ointment product works especially well to treat the rash, protect the skin, and allow it to heal. Alternatively, your pediatrician may advise you to layer zinc oxide diaper cream on top of an over-the-counter yeast cream with every diaper change.

104. I thought my baby would have soft, beautiful, clear skin, yet it seems like there's always a bump or blemish somewhere. Why is this, and what can I do?

There is an assortment of newborn rashes; although they are not serious and do resolve over time, they can throw a wrench into your plans for a baby announcement photo shoot. Here are the most common.

Erythema toxicum (also known as *E tox*): This common newborn rash typically develops on the second

or third day after birth. It tends to look quite a bit
like bug bites—the skin has several white, blister-like
bumps, with an area of redness surrounding each
blister. Erythema toxicum can occur anywhere on
the body. No one knows exactly what causes this, but
there's no need to be concerned. Once your pediatrician confirms the diagnosis, you can rest assured that
this newborn rash is harmless and usually resolves on
its own by 2 to 4 weeks of age. In the meantime, leave
the blisters alone.

**Baby acne (more accurately known as neonatal cephalic
pustulosis):** Yes, babies can get acne too! This undesirable yet relatively harmless baby rash usually shows up
3 or 4 weeks after birth and, for many babies, improves
by 2 or 3 months. Exposure to the hormones that
are transferred from mom to baby is often to blame.
Most of the time, the best treatment for baby acne is
no treatment at all. You can simply continue to gently wash your baby's skin with plain water or a mild,
fragrance-free baby wash or shampoo. In addition, ask
your pediatrician if it might help to use an over-the-
counter or prescription topical medication on specific
spots once a day for 1 or 2 days to temporarily tame
them for a special event or photo session. Don't worry—
just because your infant develops acne does not mean
he will have more acne as a teen.

Cradle cap (also known as seborrheic dermatitis):
Cradle cap is basically the baby equivalent of dandruff. These dry, flaky, and sometimes yellow and
greasy appearing patches commonly occur on the

scalp, eyebrows, and behind the ears. In its mild form, cradle cap typically is treated with mild, non-medicated baby shampoos used daily, combined with gentle brushing of the scales using a soft bristle baby brush or washcloth. Several infant cradle cap shampoos are on the market that you may wish to try. For more pronounced cases, your pediatrician may recommend using an antifungal shampoo, a small amount of adult dandruff shampoo, or 1% hydrocortisone cream or prescription steroid oil on your baby's scalp. Be careful not to get these products in a baby's eyes. While petroleum jelly products and vegetable or coconut oils (coconut oil is a popular choice and works well for baby skin and hair) may also help soften cradle cap so you can comb out flakes, if your child has a full head of hair, these products can be somewhat greasy and challenging to wash out. Olive oil is not recommended as it may increase growth of yeast and worsen cradle cap. If your baby's cradle cap is leaving you scratching your head, be sure to go over a plan of action with your pediatrician at your next well-baby examination.

105. My toddler developed a rash all over her body. She's acting normally. Do I need to bring her to the pediatrician?

Many things, including an infection (such as a virus) or contact with an irritating substance (such as soap or drool), can cause a rash, often without other symptoms.

If this is the case and she is otherwise acting normally, it's okay to keep an eye on the rash for a few days. Most rashes that have no other associated symptoms resolve on their own without treatment, sometimes before any cause can be identified.

 If the rash worsens or isn't improving within 2 or 3 days, if it begins bothering your baby, or if she develops a fever or starts acting sick, call your pediatrician.

106. My child had a fever for 3 days without any other symptoms. The fever went away, but now he has a rash. What should I do?

While it's always a good idea to touch base with your pediatrician, in most instances like this, parents don't need to do anything at all as long as their child is 3 months of age or older and is feeling all right. These symptoms are suggestive of a classic childhood viral infection known as *roseola*. Fever (temperature often 102°F [39°C] and higher) without any other symptoms can leave parents and pediatricians alike looking for answers. After about 3 days, the answer usually becomes quite clear as the fever resolves and is followed within a day or so by a telltale roseola rash (flat, pink, nonitchy spots that typically start in the center of the body and move outward to the arms and legs). By the time the rash appears, children are no longer contagious and can return—rash and all—to normal activities (eg, preschool, mommy-and-me class). The rash usually goes away on its own within 3 to 4 days.

 If your child's fever and rash don't follow this specific pattern, if the fever lasts more than 3 days, if your infant is younger than 3 months, if the rash is bothering your child, or if she looks really sick, call your pediatrician and have your child evaluated.

107.   After a week of having a stuffy, runny nose, my child has little honey-colored, crusty scabs on her face. What is this, and how do I clear it up?

It sounds like your child may have impetigo, an infection of the skin that is caused by 1 of 2 types of common bacteria (*Staphylococcus,* also known as *staph,* and *Streptococcus,* also known as *strep*) that dwell in many people's noses and on their skin. Classically, these honey-crusted sores are found on the face, often appearing during or after a cold or sinus infection. The excess nasal drainage (not to mention little fingers poking around) increases the likelihood that these nose-dwelling bacteria will spread to surrounding skin. You'll want to see your pediatrician to confirm the diagnosis and get proper treatment. Topical antibiotic ointment (such as mupirocin) is often used to clear up impetigo, but if there are many lesions, if it is spreading, or if it keeps recurring despite the use of an ointment, oral antibiotics may be needed to get rid of the infection.

108. My son has a tender, red, raised area on his leg. I'm not sure what happened, but I think it's infected. What do I do?

Any break in the skin—whether it's from a cut, a scrape, or an insect bite—has the potential to become infected. Whenever an area of skin becomes tender, warm, and red or contains pus, it is important to seek medical attention right away, because bacterial infections of the skin are serious business and can spread quickly if not evaluated and treated appropriately.

Methicillin-resistant *Staphylococcus aureus* (MRSA) is a bad bug (it's technically a type of bacteria, but it's often referred to as a *bug*, nonetheless). Like other types of staph, MRSA can live on your skin or in your nose unnoticed, until a simple scrape or scratch allows it to get through the skin's defenses, and boom, you may be faced with a bad skin infection. Infections often start out looking like a pimple or a bite and may progress rather quickly. In addition, the bacteria can stick around in your house and wreak havoc on all who enter. In the case of MRSA, the resulting skin infection is particularly difficult to treat because this type of staph is resistant to many common antibiotics used for skin infections. Close medical supervision and specific antibiotics are needed to treat MRSA. Sometimes, the infected pus needs to be drained with or without an antibiotic. To prevent infection of other family members and to get rid of any lingering bacteria from your home, your doctor may recommend some of the following for the infected person and/or all household members:

☐ Use an antibiotic ointment (such as mupirocin) in all noses in the household twice a day for 5 days.

☐ Add bleach (1 teaspoon of regular-strength bleach per gallon of water) to a bath and soak for 15 minutes twice a week. Just be sure to air out the bathroom well, especially if your child has asthma.

☐ Clean the skin with an over-the-counter antimicrobial soap (such as Hibiclens) twice a week.

☐ Wash towels, underwear, and sleepwear daily in hot water and dry them on a high-heat setting.

☐ Keep fingernails clean and short to prevent scratching and spreading.

With any skin infection, a fever can mean that bacteria have spread into the bloodstream, so call your doctor immediately. Hospitalization and administration of intravenous antibiotics may be needed.

109. My daughter has these shiny, skin-colored pimples on her chest and arms. They don't seem to be bothering her, but more and more seem to be appearing every day. What is this, and do I need to do anything?

She may have a virus called *molluscum contagiosum,* a common childhood infection spread by skin-to-skin contact. This virus usually causes small, shiny, skin-colored bumps—with a tiny, pinhole dot in the center—to appear on the skin, starting in the center of the body and spreading to the arms and legs. Occasionally, the bumps can be itchy, but usually children are not bothered by them. Molluscum contagiosum usually resolves on its own without complications, but it can take a while—sometimes a year or longer—to go away completely. If the bumps persist or are bothering your child or you, your pediatrician may apply a topical treatment in the office called *cantharidin* or recommend visiting a dermatologist for treatment. Though molluscum contagiosum is a virus, your child can still go to child care and participate in activities and classes. However, any bumps in areas that could come into contact with other people should be covered, and your daughter should take solo baths with her own towels to reduce the risk of transmitting the virus to other children.

 Call your pediatrician if your child has any molluscum contagiosum bumps near her eyes. These bumps may require a referral to an ophthalmologist (eye doctor) for close observation and management. Also, call your pediatrician if there are any signs of infection (usually from scratching), such as pain, redness, or pus.

Slather on the Sunscreen

Children have very sensitive skin and can burn easily if exposed to the sun. Even little ones with darker skin are at risk. To protect your child from an uncomfortable sunburn and skin cancer later in life, keep your child's skin covered with light clothing and keep her out of direct sunlight as much as possible. Try and limit sun exposure during the peak intensity hours, between 10 am and 4 pm. You can also purchase clothing, hats, and stroller shades with built-in sun protection or add a special laundry aid to the wash that increases the sun protection of the clothes you already own.

For babies younger than 6 months, broad-spectrum, chemical-free sunscreen with at least SPF (sun protection factor) 30 may be used on small areas of the body, such as the face and the backs of the hands, if adequate clothing and shade are not available. After 6 months of age, slather her with sunscreen 30 minutes prior to heading outdoors. Chemical-free barrier sunscreens that contain zinc oxide or titanium dioxide and are labeled as broad spectrum with SPF 30 or greater are usually best. Whichever brand you choose, test it out on your baby's back for a reaction before applying it all over. Apply sunscreen 20 to 30 minutes before going outside and reapply every 1 to 2 hours and after getting wet or sweating.

Sunglasses with ultraviolet protection can be used to shield her eyes, and a hat will protect her head. Keeping these on her can be challenging, but play a game or make fun names for them (eg, robot glasses, zookeeper hat) and be a good role model by using sun protection yourself.

Things That Make You Itch

110. What is eczema, and how do I treat it?

Eczema, or atopic dermatitis, is a chronic, allergic skin condition. It is most common in infants and young children with a family history of asthma and/or allergies. Patchy areas of skin become dry, itchy, and irritated. In more serious cases, there may also be redness, swelling, cracking, weeping, crusting, or scaling. Eczema can be triggered by any number of factors, including food, soap, detergent, fabric softener, temperature changes, sweating, or other things that irritate or dry out the skin. For some children, flare-ups are few and far between. Others may be faced with ongoing symptoms that can vary considerably in severity, ranging from mild to quite widespread.

While eczema itself is a condition that can't technically be cured, children often outgrow it. In the meantime, it is entirely possible to treat eczema and prevent its symptoms from recurring. First, stay away from anything that you know causes the rash in your child. Often, though, it isn't one specific thing but a combination of factors that can trigger the eczema. Decreasing all allergenic or skin-drying substances in your child's environment can help and is not as daunting as it may seem. For example, use laundry detergent that is free of perfume and dye. Steer clear of fabric softeners; they are not recommended for children with eczema. Daily bathing is recommended for children with eczema, and soaps should be avoided because they can dry the skin. Instead, use a mild, unscented body wash. After your child's bath, gently pat his skin dry and slather an ointment or thick cream all over. It's best to apply the moisturizer within 3 minutes of getting out of the bath, before the water evaporates and dries the skin even more.

Use ointment or cream on your little one twice a day to keep the skin hydrated and help prevent bad, uncomfortable flare-ups. Make sure your child's skin is wet when applying the ointment or cream, as this will help it get absorbed. You can use a spritzer bottle filled with water on your child's skin prior to application of the ointments or cream.

When your child's eczema worsens, talk to your pediatrician, as there are many steroids of various strengths and nonsteroid creams that can be used on a regular basis or on an as-needed basis. If your child is up all night itching and scratching (which can worsen an infection, as well as delay healing), your pediatrician may recommend an antihistamine as well.

 If you see any oozing, pus, or increasing redness and tenderness of the skin, or if your child develops a fever, call your pediatrician—these can all be signs of a skin infection.

111. Yikes! My daughter broke out in an itchy, welt-like rash (hives) while we were eating at a restaurant. What should I do?

Whenever a child seems to be reacting to something she ate or came into contact with, be sure that the rash is not accompanied by any more concerning signs of an allergic reaction, such as wheezing, trouble swallowing or drooling, or facial swelling. Once you've determined that you're only dealing with an itchy rash with areas of raised red bumps, sometimes with pale centers, it is quite likely that your child has hives. Hives may appear all over the body almost instantly (or within a few hours) after eating or touching something specific. Or hives may appear on one area of the body, disappear, and reappear later somewhere else. Foods (such as milk, eggs, nuts, and shellfish), medication (such as penicillin), or a bee sting can all cause hives. In addition, hives can accompany a number of viral infections. Although frequently the cause cannot be identified, make a list of everything that your child ate (such as food or medication) or touched several hours before the rash appeared, as well as any recent bee stings or illnesses. Take the list to your pediatrician to help identify any potential cause of the hives, and—often more pressing in the moment—discuss how to take the itch out of the situation.

Hives can be super itchy and make your child feel miserable. To help treat the hives and offer some relief from the itching, your pediatrician may recommend an oral antihistamine (like over-the-counter cetirizine). In cases in which hives keep showing up, your pediatrician may recommend using an antihistamine daily for a few days to help prevent and control the hives. Nonsedating antihistamines (such as cetirizine) won't make your child drowsy and are now recommended over diphenhydramine. If your infant or child has allergies, it is wise to be prepared and have an antihistamine on hand at all times, just in case.

 Allergic reactions that cause trouble breathing can quickly become life-threatening. If your child starts wheezing, has trouble swallowing, or develops any swelling of the lips, face, tongue, throat, or neck, it is important to seek medical care immediately at the emergency department or by calling 911. Talk to your pediatrician about whether a referral to an allergist is needed to determine the cause of the reaction and assess your child's risk of having more reactions in the future.

112.   Ughhh! We seem to have head lice. How do I get rid of it?

No doubt about it, those pesky little critters can be a pain for parents and children. It doesn't mean you aren't keeping your child clean enough, as lice seem to prefer attaching themselves to clean hair. Unfortunately, lice can spread relatively easily from one child to the next because lice can crawl (but not fly or jump) from head to head and are commonly transferred by simply sharing hats and brushes. That said, most cases of head lice can be treated relatively easily. Try using over-the-counter lice shampoo applied to a dry scalp and hair, and leave it on for as long as recommended in the package directions. Finally, comb out every nit (the tiny whitish-gray eggs) from your child's head—this can be very time consuming if there is a lot of hair! Recomb your child's hair every few days, checking for lice and nits, and repeat the process with lice shampoo 1 week after the initial treatment. There are also salons and in-home lice removal companies that can help treat and pick out each and every louse if you prefer.

To prevent lice, teach kids not to share hats, combs, hairbands, and brushes. Also, don't pile sweatshirts and jackets on top of each other at school (hang them up individually on hooks or the backs of chairs), since lice can crawl from hoodie to hoodie. For girls with long hair, keeping their hair pulled back in a ponytail or braid can also help prevent catching lice from good friends who tend to hang out in close contact, with their long hair touching their friends' hair.

 Call your pediatrician if you're not having luck eliminating the lice, as there are prescription-strength shampoos available.

Got Pinworms?

Pinworms, although not fun to find, are essentially harmless. They look like little whitish-gray threads, popping up on a child's bottom (on the skin around the anus, to be exact), usually at night. Symptoms include nighttime itching of the bottom or even the vaginal area in girls. Treatment consists of an over-the-counter or prescription pinworm medication (a chewable or liquid medication), taken once and then repeated in 2 weeks. Your pediatrician may also advise treating other family members. Wash all clothes and bedding in hot water to reduce the risk of repeat infection.

Birthmarks

113. My baby has a birthmark. What is it, and will it go away?

Some birthmarks will disappear, some will fade, and some will stay with you. Here are some facts about the most common birthmarks.

Stork bite or angel kiss (nevus simplex): Remember when someone in your childhood told you that the stork brought new babies into the world? The term *stork bite* comes from this fable, and the birthmark looks like a flat, pink or red mark on the back of the neck. The same type of birthmark on the forehead or eyelids is often called an *angel kiss*. These harmless birthmarks may become more noticeable when a baby cries or during a bath because of an increase in body temperature and blood flow. Their presence is often short-lived, as most fade with time and are hardly noticeable by 4 or 5 years of age.

Hemangioma: This type of birthmark is also red but often looks more like a blood-red, raised, strawberry-type lesion. Made up of a cluster of tiny blood vessels, hemangiomas often become bigger and more pronounced before getting better. That's because hemangiomas typically grow during the first few months to a year after birth and then begin to shrink and fade (involute) from the center out. By the age of 5 years, about 50% of hemangiomas will have disappeared. By the age of 10 years, 90% of hemangiomas will be gone. These birthmarks often do not need to be treated or removed unless they are located in areas where they may interfere with important functions, such as over the eyes (where they may interfere with vision) or in the mouth or throat (where they can interfere with breathing or eating). These types of birthmarks are also removed for cosmetic reasons or because they are located in easily bumped areas, since hemangiomas are prone to bleeding. Topical or oral medication (usually prescribed by a specialist) is now commonly used to shrink hemangiomas.

Congenital dermal melanocytosis or "slate-gray" spots (formerly called Mongolian spots): Often confused with a bruise early on, this birthmark looks bluish-gray and is most commonly located on a child's back or buttocks. These spots are more common in darker-skinned babies. They tend to fade by school age, and they are not dangerous.

CHAPTER 11

Child Care

During your pregnancy is a good time to begin thinking about whether you are going to want help caring for your baby. Will you be staying home with your baby? Or will you be taking maternity leave and going back to work (either in person or virtually)? Do you have a partner, spouse, or relative who can help you? Do you want to hire a baby nurse, doula, or nanny? Do you want to look at child care options in your area? These questions aren't meant to make you stressed, but beginning to think about all your options sooner rather than later will help you make the best decision for your child and family. It often does take a village—or at least another set of hands at some point—to help raise a child.

114. Can I hire somebody to help me care for my baby after delivery?

Of course! Some moms like to have an extra set of hands and a little help after delivery, and there's nothing wrong with that. This can be especially helpful if you had a C-section or a complicated delivery, if you don't have a partner to help you, if you have other young children at home who also need care, or if you or your partner must return to a job quickly after the birth. It's a good idea to hire someone who is specially trained in newborn care (including infant CPR [cardiopulmonary resuscitation]) and breastfeeding. Good options are a baby nurse, a doula (who may also be able to help during labor and delivery), and/or a lactation consultant. Some of these individuals may work nights only, or days only, for a limited amount of time after delivery—such as days, weeks, or months—and then move on to help another mom after delivery. Make sure you take the opportunity to learn from these specialists while they are with you, so that when they go, you are able to continue caring for your baby.

115.   When should I begin looking for child care for my baby, and what should I look for?

It's a good idea to start thinking about your options during pregnancy. If you are working, ask your employer about their maternity leave policy. Find out if you qualify for short-term disability and/or leave granted by the Family and Medical Leave Act (FMLA). This can help you decide how long you may be able to stay home with your baby before needing to return to work. Then, think about whether you'd like somebody to care for your child in your home or if you'd like to drop your child off at an in-home child care or a child care facility. There isn't a right or wrong answer—it totally depends on your desire and your budget.

To find a qualified and loving child care provider, ask everyone you know for suggestions: Ask your friends, neighbors, colleagues, and even your pediatrician. I found all my nannies and sitters from friends who didn't need child care help anymore. Getting a personal recommendation from somebody you trust is fantastic. It's also often a good idea to use a child care agency; there is a fee, but that way, the nanny or child care provider you hire is thoroughly vetted and has undergone a background check. If the nanny or provider doesn't work out, the service will send somebody else to your house to replace her. The next few questions cover some pros and cons to think about as you decide what type of child care is best for your family.

116. I think I'd like to have somebody help me care for my baby in my home. What are my options?

Some parents prefer to have somebody come into their home or even live with them to help care for their new baby and/or older children. Most commonly, a nanny or an au pair will provide care for your child or children in your own home.

Nanny

A nanny typically comes to your home to care for your baby or older child. This is often a more

expensive option than child care, but there can be
many benefits, such as your child's getting to know
one trusted adult who cares for her and creating a
routine of having your child, eat, nap, and play at
home. You also don't have to wake your kids up
early and get them dressed, fed, and out the door
before work in the morning. The biggest benefit to
hiring a nanny that I see as a pediatrician is that
your child is usually exposed to fewer illnesses since
he isn't around other potentially sick kids. The hard
part may be if your nanny gets sick and isn't able
to work. If this happens, you may need another
helping hand.

Au Pair

An au pair is a young adult who lives in your home
as part of a government-regulated international
cultural exchange program and cares for your
children for a certain number of hours a week.
The cost is often less than that of a nanny, but
you, as the host family, must provide a bedroom,
bathroom, car, and auto insurance for the au pair.
The benefits are that your family is exposed to a
different culture and often a new language, and the
au pair's hours are typically flexible, so you can get
up early for work or go out at night while the au pair
cares for your child. The cons for some families are
that the au pair can only stay for a year or two at
a time before she must return home to her country
of origin.

117. What's the difference between an in-home child care and a facility child care?

Child care can be a wonderful option for families who are looking for part-time or full-time care for their child. Generally speaking, child cares are located either in somebody else's home or a larger child care facility. Which option you choose may depend on your family's needs and desires, as well as location—hopefully, one close to your home or work.

In-Home Child Care

An in-home child care is a good option for families looking for a small, personal setting with a limited number of other children. Also, in-home child care is often less expensive than other child care options. Make sure you thoroughly research the in-home child care you are considering and talk with parents whose children attend that child care as well. Find out if the provider is licensed and if other caregivers or people will be in the home during the time your child will be there. Take a tour of the home and see how many infants and/or toddlers are attending, where and how everyone naps (sleep safety is important to decrease the risk of sudden infant death syndrome [SIDS]), and how kids are cared for, played with, and fed. Also, ask about their hours, what happens if you need to drop your child off early or pick him up late, and their policy for when a child is sick. A strict policy of keeping your child at home if he is sick is good to prevent other children from catching illnesses, but it can also make it challenging for you to get to work if your child only has the sniffles.

Child Care Facility

There are many licensed child care facilities that range in price, size, and structure. Some facilities accept infants and then transition them as they get older into toddler and preschool classes. They have curricula for how they play and what they teach at various ages, along with set hours, although these hours usually include early-morning drop-off and late pickup options. I suggest that you take a tour of each facility and look up, down, and all around for cleanliness and space to play, both inside and outside. Ask questions about the child care providers, daily routines, sleep schedules, cleaning protocols, and play and feeding arrangements. Ask how the facility keeps records on infant schedules, what happens when one of their child care providers is out sick, and what their sick policy is for keeping potentially infectious kids at home. Get a feel for each facility and whether it's a place where you would feel comfortable dropping off your child, knowing she will receive loving, appropriate care. And remember to have a backup option for when your little one gets sick, can't attend child care, and needs to stay home.

Dr. Tanya's Tip

Ask the "What If" Questions

When interviewing a child care provider, ask about their experience, references, price, hours, flexibility, communication during the day (notes, photos, or videos of child?), and CPR training, as well as how the children will nap (sleep on back in bare crib) and how the provider will feed your child (in terms of healthy, appropriate food choices).

However, you will often learn the most by asking the "what if" questions: What will you do if my baby won't nap? What if he cries? What if he won't eat? What if he has a fever? What if he throws up? What if a child tests positive for COVID, RSV (respiratory syncytial virus), or influenza? What happens if the power goes out? What will you do if somebody knocks at the door while you're watching my child? What will you do if you run out of milk? What happens if I have an emergency at work and can't pick up my child on time?

By thinking and talking about all the "what if" scenarios that might worry you while you are away from your child, you can find out about the child care provider's problem-solving ability, personality, and strategy with regard to how they will care for your child. By asking these questions, you will also get them thinking ahead of time about how to safely navigate a variety of situations.

118.   Can I still exclusively breastfeed if my baby is going to child care?

Of course! It may take a little prep work, but it's totally doable. Start pumping and offering your baby a bottle at least once a day at 2 to 4 weeks of age (for more information on pumping, refer to question 21 in chapter 2, Breastfeeding). If you pump and store enough milk for 1 extra feeding a day, you can create a supply of stored breast milk, as well as teach your baby to easily drink from both breast and bottle. If possible, nurse your baby in the morning and at night, or when baby is with you. While your baby is away in child care, you can pump milk for the next day's bottles (pump if you can at every missed feed) to be given to your baby at child care. The extra supply you have at home will ensure that you have enough milk for days when you don't pump quite as much or when you are away for longer than expected and your baby needs more to drink. You can transport breast milk in a cooler bag to child care and pick up any used bottles afterward. Ask your child care provider about any specific requirements they have for labeling and storing breast milk.

119.   My son is getting over a cold. When can he return to child care or preschool or attend a birthday party or other event?

Generally speaking, he can be around other kids once his fever has been gone for 24 hours (without fever-reducing medication) and he's feeling better. If your child has been prescribed an antibiotic for any reason, he should receive the medication for at least 24 hours before being around other children. If he's vomiting, having massive diarrhea, or coughing up a storm, obviously he should rest at home and not be around other kids until these symptoms improve. Often, it's the milder symptoms (such as a slight runny nose and cough) that leave parents wondering what to do. Only you can make that game-day decision, but be considerate of others. Before you take your child out, think to yourself, "Would I want another child with the same symptoms to be around my son?" Always check with your child care or preschool; they may have specific guidelines for when previously sick children can return, especially during a pandemic or an outbreak.

Child Care Cooties

Because young children are constantly touching everything and putting their hands in their mouths, they do tend to share illnesses quickly in a child care setting. Even with strict rules that keep sick kids at home, kids are often contagious before they have symptoms, so it's virtually impossible to keep a child care facility with many kids completely illness free (the same goes for homes with several kids). Start to teach your child fun and proper handwashing techniques at an early age and practice frequently. For more information on specific illnesses your child may catch, how to treat them, and when you need to see your pediatrician or call her in the middle of the night, refer to chapter 8, Coughs, Colds, and More.

120. How do I know when my child is ready for preschool, and how do I choose a preschool?

If you are eager for your child to learn new things, meet other children the same age, and broaden her horizons, you may be ready to send her to preschool. But is she ready? Every toddler is different, but some indicators that she is ready for preschool are that she can follow directions (most of the time), she enjoys sitting and listening to books and music, she likes to meet new kids and play with others (or at least play next to others), she can adjust to leaving your side, and she can go at least 4 hours without napping. Even preschools that have naptime usually schedule it for after lunch at noon or 1 pm. Some preschools require kids to be potty-trained, while others don't and may even help with the potty-training process. Many preschools have extended hours for working parents, while others do not.

Ask around or search online for preschools in your neighborhood. Check with your local community centers, churches, and temples as well. Depending on where you live, there may be waiting lists that are months or years long. Take a few tours of the preschool facilities and get a feeling for the environment. Do the children seem happy? Do the classrooms and bathrooms seem clean? Is there outdoor playtime? Are the teachers credentialed and/or certified? Are they warm and caring? Do they know how to interact with and teach young children? Do they have a curriculum for each age group? Even play-based preschools can usually tell you the kind of age-appropriate activities they have for each class. What is the teacher-to-student ratio? Are the preschool grounds secure? What is the preschool staff's strategy for keeping track of all students and visitors?

If you decide it's time to send your child to preschool, make sure you prepare her ahead of time. Talk about how she is old enough now to go to a big girl school and how exciting it will be, run through everything that will happen during the day, and be sure to remind her that you will see her after school. It's also important to note that while preschool can be a wonderful experience for young children and help prepare them for kindergarten, it isn't a must. As long as a child has a caring adult to enrich her in whatever environment she is in, she should be ready to start prekindergarten, transitional kindergarten, or regular kindergarten on time.

CHAPTER 12

Ingestions, Injuries, and First Aid

ometimes injuries happen. It would be nice if we could protect our children from danger 100% of the time, but that's just not realistic. To add insult to injury, kids climb and jump when we'd like them to sit still, and they touch and eat things that we thought were out of their reach. Fortunately, most of the time it isn't serious, but some injuries can be life-threatening. Do your best to protect your children—always buckle them up in properly installed car seats, baby proof your house, and keep a close eye on your little ones when you are out. Even with the most vigilant care and the best baby-proofing skills, injuries may still happen, so it is important for you to be prepared and know what to do should the need arise.

Dr. Tanya's Tip

Emergency Information

Keep the following information on the front of your refrigerator, near a house phone, and in your cell phone:

☐ Your child's name, birth date, and current weight

☐ Your child's regular medications, with dosage and directions

☐ Any allergies or medical conditions your child has

☐ Your contact information (work and cell phone numbers)

☐ Your house address and phone number

☐ Your pediatrician's name and contact information

☐ Your preferred hospital and pharmacy, with phone numbers

☐ A photo of your child's health insurance card

☐ Another emergency adult contact

☐ Poison control contact information (1-800-222-1222)

Ingestions

121. My child ate berries off of a plant, swallowed a pill I accidentally dropped, drank dishwasher soap, or (fill in the blank). What do I do?

Repeat after me . . . *call Poison Control at* 1-800-222-1222. Always keep the number for poison control handy (on your fridge, near a house phone, and in your cell phone) for such emergencies. This number is so helpful, even your pediatrician uses it! If you have any information about what your child ingested (such as the color and shape of a pill, as well as any markings on it), let Poison Control know.

Or, if you can, take a photo of an object identical to what your child ate and text or email it to your pediatrician. If you're not able to get a photo, then give your pediatrician as much information as you can. He will instruct you on what to do. It is no longer recommended to give syrup of ipecac to make your child throw up—sometimes, this can cause further harm.

 Of course, if your child is not acting well or if the situation is a true emergency, call 911. If you have any other questions or concerns, call your pediatrician.

122. I think my child swallowed a coin! What should I do?

As long as your child is acting normally (ie, he can breathe and talk and drink fine), try not to panic. Most coins smaller than a quarter will pass right through him without getting stuck. Touch base with your pediatrician, who may advise you to check your child's stool for a few days until you find the coin. If it doesn't come out, a doctor may have to go looking for it. A simple x-ray can show the doctor exactly where the coin is and help her decide whether a specialist needs to retrieve it. If your child is in diapers, it's easier to search a dirty diaper for loose change. If he is toilet trained, have him poop on a paper plate or loosely place plastic wrap inside the toilet to catch your child's poop. Isn't parenting fun?

 If your child is choking, having trouble breathing, drooling, or in pain (in the mouth, throat, or tummy), call 911. If your child has swallowed quarters or anything larger, any size batteries or magnets, or sharp objects like pins or tacks, call your doctor and head to the emergency department immediately! If you aren't sure what your child swallowed, call your pediatrician for advice.

Up the Nose or in the Ear

Kids love to put beads, peas, and you-name-it up their noses or in their ears. I can't tell you how many of these items I've retrieved. Placing objects up the nose or in the mouth can be serious because, if they're inhaled, they can interfere with a child's breathing. It is less dangerous if an object is placed in the ear because the eardrum prevents the object from going too far inside. But wherever Sammy hid his veggies, they must be removed to avoid complications, such as bleeding or infection.

If your child inserts an object into his nose or his ear, call your pediatrician as soon as possible to find out if she can see your child or if she wants you to go straight to urgent care or the emergency department to have the object removed.

Injuries

123. Help! My baby fell off the couch, and I think she hit her head. What should I do?

Even though newborns rarely roll over on their own, they can wiggle and squirm, which is how they some-how manage to fall off couches and changing tables when parents turn away . . . even for just a moment. So, after the loud thud is heard throughout the house, how do you know if your baby is truly injured? Usually, a baby will cry immediately and then calm down when picked up and comforted by a parent. Once she is calm, look your child over for any visibly injured areas, use your hand to gently press all over her head and body, looking for any tender areas that make her cry. If any-thing seems to hurt or if the initial crying persists, your baby should be evaluated right away.

Luckily, most falls, whether they involve beds or couches or walking or running, do not result in serious injury. The most common cause for concern is head trauma, and unless you saw your toddler fall, it may not be apparent if she hit her head. If your child loses consciousness after the fall, she needs to be evaluated as soon as possible, so take her to the nearest emer-gency department. If she cries for a moment and then continues playing, your pediatrician may ask you to closely observe her at home. Check your child's scalp. Large, goose egg–sized bumps are typically a sign of injury on the outside of the skull, not the inside, where the brain is. If your child will let you, apply ice (or a bag of frozen peas) wrapped in a cloth for a few minutes to help soothe the pain and decrease the swelling. Repeat this every 4 hours as needed. As long as your child is acting all right, your doctor will probably say there's no need to wake her up throughout the night to check on her.

 Call 911 if your baby or child loses consciousness or is seriously injured. Otherwise, call your pediatrician and explain what happened. The doctor may want to see your child in the office or have you take her to the emergency department, especially for the following reasons:

- ☐ The fall occurred from a height of more than approximately 3 feet.
- ☐ Your child is not responding as she usually does.
- ☐ Your child is continuously crying.
- ☐ Your child is vomiting.
- ☐ Your child complains of a severe headache.
- ☐ Your child is lethargic.
- ☐ Your child is overly sleepy.
- ☐ Your child is not talking or walking as usual.
- ☐ Later, your child is not feeding or acting as she usually does.

To prevent falls, buckle the safety strap around your child when she is on the changing table, don't leave her alone on a bed or a couch, and never put her in a bouncy seat or a car seat on an elevated surface, such as a table top or countertop.

Call your pediatrician and go to the emergency department if your child begins complaining of a severe headache or if she cries uncontrollably, vomits, is too sleepy, is not responding as usual, or is talking, walking, or acting abnormally. Also, if your child has a cut that won't stop bleeding after applying direct pressure for 5 minutes, call your pediatrician.

124.   My toddler was running, and he tripped and fell. Now he is crying and won't walk. How do I know if he broke something?

You can't know for sure. Even doctors can't always tell if there is a break without obtaining an x-ray. If the injury happens during office hours, you can always call your doctor to schedule an appointment. More often than not, such injuries seem to happen after hours or on the weekend. Before you rush to the emergency department, give the situation a few minutes and try to comfort your child. Once he calms down, you can give him an appropriate dose of ibuprofen (Motrin or Advil) or acetaminophen (Tylenol) and apply ice to the injury if he'll let you. If there is an obvious deformity where the injury occurred or if he continues to scream in pain and refuses to stand or walk, it's best to have him evaluated (you're probably warming up your car as you read this, anyway). If your child seems to be fine or if it's late at night, it's okay to wait until the next morning for the injury to be evaluated. Your child may get better and start walking again on his own.

By the following day, if your child is walking around normally, don't worry about it. Your toddler probably just had a minor injury (not a fracture, or break) that has already healed. If he's still limping or seems to be in pain, make an appointment with your pediatrician. The doctor may obtain an x-ray to look for a "toddler fracture" (see the next question). It isn't a serious condition, but your child's leg will need to be immobilized—usually with a cast for a few weeks—to heal properly.

125. My toddler has been limping for a few days or refusing to walk on 2 legs. I don't remember him getting hurt. What should I do?

A common toddler injury is called a "toddler fracture." It can happen when toddlers slide down off of the couch (my youngest son fractured his leg this way on my husband's watch), slide down a slide, or jump in a "bounce house" and land or get their foot caught with a slight twist in their leg. It's usually a low-impact injury that causes a slight spiral break in the bottom of the larger leg bone (the tibia). Sometimes, toddlers will cry when this happens, and other times they won't. You may see some swelling of the shin, ankle, or foot. Often, they don't seem bothered by it except when trying to walk on it, and they will quickly learn how to avoid the pain by limping or crawling. Casting performed by an orthopedist is needed for the bone to heal

properly, so a visit to your pediatrician or a specialist to obtain an x-ray is needed.

As long as your toddler is happy and not in pain, it's
okay to wait until the following morning to have him
examined and obtain an x-ray.

 If your toddler has a fever, is crying because of his pain level,
or looks sick, call your pediatrician right away, as he may
have something more serious than a simple toddler fracture.

126. I picked up my child by her arms, and now she's holding one arm down by her side. She won't move her arm, and she cries when I try to touch it. Did I break something?

This common injury is called a *nursemaid elbow.*
Any sudden upward pull on a child's arm can cause
the elbow to come out of the joint, which is called a
dislocation. Luckily, your pediatrician should be able
to put the arm back into place in the office by using
a simple arm maneuver. (After I fix such an injury, I
like to place a lollipop in the hand of the previously
injured arm and leave the room. I check back in 5
minutes, and the child is always happily licking the
lollipop, which means the arm is now fine.) Although
there are no long-term complications from this injury
because the ligaments are slightly stretched temporarily, some toddlers may be prone to elbow dislocation. As kids get older, the ligaments in their elbow

naturally tighten so they are less prone to getting a
nursemaid elbow.

If a child experiences this injury, Mommy and
Daddy need to take a break from playing helicopter
with the child. In the future, pick your child up
under the arms or around the chest to avoid injuring
her arms.

127. My child is crying and rubbing his eye, and it looks a little red. I'm worried something got into his eye, but I can't see anything. What should I do?

Eye injuries, while all too common during childhood,
should always be taken seriously. If you suspect that
your child has something in his eye (eg, sand, an eye-
lash, soap), the first thing to do is gently splash clean
water or saline into the eye. If that doesn't seem to
relieve his discomfort, you may need to do a thorough
check of the eye (if he will let you!). This may include
pulling down the lower eyelid and flipping the upper
eyelid back, in addition to checking the white part of
the eye. If you see something, you can sweep it away
with a clean cotton swab or try to rinse it out with
clean water or saline. If you still don't see anything, if
you are uncomfortable with checking your child's eye,
or if you are concerned that whatever got into his eye
may have scratched part of the eye (called a *corneal
abrasion*), call your pediatrician or go to an ophthalmologist (eye doctor) or the emergency department.

A corneal abrasion can occur from any particulate matter getting in the eye, an eye getting poked with a stick or finger, or even a powerful squirt in the eye from a water gun.

 If you are concerned that your child's eye came into contact with any liquid that contains chemicals such as acids or bases (eg, lye, baking soda, or ammonia), immediately start rinsing the affected eye with lots of water or saline. Continue rinsing the eye on the way to the emergency department, as these substances can cause chemical burns to the eye that can permanently affect your child's vision.

Home First-Aid Kit

Many trips to the pediatrician's office or emergency department can be avoided by keeping a fully stocked first-aid kit at home. Although there are many premade first-aid kits that can be purchased at your local pharmacy or online, make sure they have the following components. Or you can make or add your own!

☐ Bandages of various sizes, gauze, tape, and other supplies for bandaging up "owies"
☐ Disposable gloves and/or hand sanitizer to disinfect your hands
☐ Scissors

Continued on next page

☐ Tweezers for removing splinters or bug stingers

☐ Thermometer

☐ Cold and/or heat packs

☐ Small flashlight

☐ Bottle of water (to clean those "owies" or to hydrate your little one if he looks dehydrated)

☐ Acetaminophen or ibuprofen (see the dosing chart in chapter 7) for fever or pain

☐ Antihistamine (such as cetirizine) for itching or allergies

☐ Cortisone cream for insect bites or itchy rashes

☐ Antibiotic ointment for cuts and scrapes

☐ Wound-numbing spray for minor burns or cuts

☐ Any medications that your child (a) takes regularly or on an as-needed basis or (b) may need for an emergency, such as asthma medication or an epinephrine pen

Keep your first-aid kit in a place that is easy for an adult to reach (and easy for a babysitter to find), but out of a child's reach.

Car Seats

Automobile crashes are the No. 1 cause of death in children. While you can't control others on the road, you can make sure that your family always buckles up safely. Don't forget to have your car seat checked by a trained professional. Proper installation and use are key to protecting your little one during a crash.

128. Which car seat is best for my child? I'm so confused.

You're not alone. With so many choices available, there isn't one seat that is the "best" or "safest," so car seat confusion is common. The best seat is simply the one that fits your child's size and age, is correctly installed, and is used properly every time you drive. Have your car seat installation checked by a trained professional. Many police departments and fire stations have trained child passenger safety technicians who will check your car seat. Or you can visit NHTSA.gov to help find options near you.

If you haven't already bought a car safety seat for your newborn, you will need one to safely transport your new baby home from the hospital. Many parents like to start with an infant-only car seat because the base can be left in the car (you can buy extra bases if you have more than 1 car), and the seat clicks in and out of the base for easy transport of your little one. Most hospitals require new parents to show that they have a car safety seat for their infant's first ride home, so it is best to purchase and install the seat ahead of time. The car seat must be rear-facing and installed in the back seat. If this is your first child (and she will be in the only car seat in your car), the rear center seat is recommended for her car seat placement if you can get a tight installation in that position. However, the center position in some cars is narrow or uneven, and LATCH straps are usually not allowed in the center position. If you cannot install the base tightly in the center rear seat or if you need to put 2 car seats in the back, the most comfortable fit may be to have 1 on each side of the car.

As your infant grows, he will outgrow the rear-facing car seat, which leaves many parents wondering what to buy next. (Check the weight and height limit on the car seat label to know exactly when your child will need a new car seat.) A convertible car seat is usually the next step. As the name implies, this can be used in a rear-facing position now; when your child is older, the car seat can be turned around to become a forward-facing seat.

Safety experts and the American Academy of Pediatrics recommend that children should remain rear-facing until at least age 2 years or whenever they reach the maximum weight or height allowed by the car seat. By law, many states require that rear-facing car seats be used until age 2 years. It is not necessary to move a child to a forward-facing position to give him leg room; rear-facing seats are more comfortable than you would imagine, and leg injuries are very rare when children are in the rear-facing position. There's no question that the rear-facing position is definitely the safest way for a child to ride.

Dr. Tanya's Tip

Babyproofing

Children can be quite the explorers! As soon as your little one starts reaching out and grabbing things on her own, it is a good idea to start thinking about babyproofing your home. Here are some tips to keeping your child safe at home.

First things first, get down on your hands and knees and crawl around your living space to identify electrical sockets, small objects, or loose articles your explorer may find.

Use plug protectors in all outlets.

Make sure all cleaners, soaps, laundry detergents, medicines, and small objects are kept in secured places that are out of your child's reach.

Put gates at the top and bottom of any stairs to avoid falls.

Make sure all drapery cords and cords for window blinds are out of reach. Loose cords can strangle children.

Keep nightlights away from drapes or bedding, where they could start a fire. Consider using cool nightlights that do not get hot.

Secure all windows by locking them and/or putting up guards to prevent your child from falling out.

If your home has a pool, make sure it is surrounded on all 4 sides by a fence at least 4 feet high, with a self-closing, self-latching gate.

Other things you can do to keep everyone safe include placing working smoke and carbon dioxide detectors through-

Continued on next page

out your home, keeping a working fire extinguisher somewhere in your kitchen, and making sure your water heater
is set to a maximum temperature of no more than 120°F to
avoid burns. Also, a home is safest without firearms. If you
must have a gun, make sure that it is stored unloaded and
locked in a safe or with a trigger lock and that bullets are
locked away in another separate place.

Cuts, Scrapes, and Bites . . . Oh My!

129. How do I know if my child needs stitches?

Cuts and scrapes are common injuries for active kiddos. A cut that is deep, has gaping skin, or won't stop
bleeding after 10 minutes of applying constant, direct
pressure may need stitches to close the wound. On
some areas of the body, a doctor can apply a special
glue (like super glue, only safe for skin) or staples
(again, specially made for skin—usually the scalp) to
keep a wound closed, instead of stitches. Bring your
child's immunization records with you to the doctor; she may need a tetanus shot, depending on what
caused the injury and when she received her last
tetanus booster.

 If you think your child has a cut that needs to be medically
closed, call your pediatrician to find out if this can be done
in the office or if you need to go to an urgent care center, an

emergency department, or a plastic surgeon. Don't wait too long—it's often best to take care of a cut within 4 to 8 hours of the injury. Signs of infection, such as fever, redness, pain, swelling, or pus, also need to be evaluated as soon as possible.

Getting Splinters Out

Clean the area around the splinter well, and let it soak in warm, soapy water. Apply an over-the-counter numbing cream. You can then try to remove the splinter with tweezers by grabbing the protruding end and pulling gently. If you can't get the splinter out, you can wait a few days to see if it works itself out.

 If the splinter is deep or doesn't come out soon on its own, or if there are signs of infection, such as redness, swelling, oozing, or pain, please be sure to see your pediatrician.

130. An insect bit/stung my son, and now the area is swollen and red. What should I do?

Ouch! First, look to see if there is any visible stinger. If so, remove it by gently scraping horizontally across the skin with the edge of a credit card or a clean fingernail. Wash the area with soap and water and apply ice or a cool compress to help decrease the pain and swelling. You can also give your child an appropriate dose of ibuprofen (if the child is older than 6 months) or acetaminophen for the pain. If the bite or sting seems itchy, you can try applying a topical anti-itch medication (like hydrocortisone cream or calamine lotion) or give your child an appropriate dose of an antihistamine, like cetirizine. Ask your pediatrician if you are unsure about the proper dose for your child.

 If there are any signs of a secondary bacterial skin infection from a bite or sting, such as increasing redness, pain, drainage, or pus, see your pediatrician, because treatment with an antibiotic may be needed. In addition, if there are any signs of a serious allergic reaction to the bite or sting, such as trouble breathing or swallowing, seek medical attention immediately!

131. My toddler was accidentally bitten by another child, a dog, or other animal. What do I need to do?

If your child is bleeding from the bite, apply firm pressure continuously for 5 minutes or until the bleeding stops. Then, wash the wound well but gently with soap and water.

Contact your pediatrician for any bite that breaks the skin, as she will need to find out if your child is protected against tetanus and, in the case of an animal bite, if there is any concern that your child needs protection against rabies. In addition, your pediatrician may recommend antibiotics, depending on the type of bite and the location, to prevent infection. Antibiotics are often prescribed to prevent infection from a dog or other animal or human bites, especially if deep.

 Call your pediatrician right away if the wound doesn't stop bleeding after applying firm pressure for 10 minutes (see question 129 for when cuts need medical attention), if the wound has jagged edges, or if your child is in severe pain.

132.   I found a tick on my child. Do I need to worry about Lyme disease?

Try not to panic. Ticks can transmit infection only after they've firmly attached themselves to the skin for at least 12 to 48 hours. A tiny, round tick that is walking on the skin or is easily removed has not yet attached to your child. Therefore, the tick is not yet capable of transmitting disease.

If the tick has latched itself onto your child, however, you should remove it as soon as possible. Gently grasp it with tweezers, as close to the skin as possible, and pull it straight out. You can place the tick in a zipper bag or other container submerged in rubbing alcohol to show your pediatrician, or take a photo of it and properly dispose of it (flush down the toilet or wrap in tape and throw away). Then, wash the area with soap and water and apply antibiotic ointment.

Be sure to check your child from head to toe to look for any more hidden ticks, because ticks can carry diseases, such as Lyme disease and others.

 Keep an eye on your child for 1 month after receiving a tick bite. If he isn't feeling well, if he looks sick, or if he develops a rash (usually at the site of the bite) or fever, call your pediatrician. When detected early, Lyme disease and other infections from ticks can be effectively treated with antibiotics.

CHAPTER 13

Growing Up

Every new thing your child does, from her first smile to her first step, is exciting and monumental. You may quickly realize, though, that your little one's timing may not be exactly the same as that of other children the same age. As a parent, it is only natural to compare your child to others. No matter how many times you are told to resist the urge to compare, you just can't. I won't pretend I can convince you to stop, but I will attempt to ease your mind by reassuring you that each and every child is unique. You will always meet a parent whose child got her first tooth, took her first steps, said her first word, used the potty on her own, and sat quietly in circle time and listened before yours was even close to becoming ready. That's okay.

Keeping that in mind, I hope you will appreciate every moment and milestone your own infant or toddler reaches and continue to play an active role in her development. I'm not going to sugarcoat it—there will be good days and bad days. But each day is a new day, full of new opportunities for learning and growing.

Growth

133. What is the best way to talk to my baby?

Start talking to your baby on day 1. Language development starts very early in life, even during the first few
months. More than 80% of a baby's brain is formed in
the first 3 years. The more you speak to your baby, the
better. No matter what language you speak, as long as
your baby is hearing properly spoken words on a daily
basis, he will develop good language skills. Some "baby
talk" is inevitable, since your baby will of course be the
cutest little thing, and you'll want to make him smile
and laugh. But make sure you also speak to him like an
older child who can talk and respond to you. Talk to
your baby about anything and everything. Talk about
your day, talk about what you are doing at that moment,
tell him a story, describe your environment, ask him
questions (even though he can't answer, it's good for
him to hear you), and talk to him about anything else
you can think of. Start reading to your baby early on; a
good time to read is at bedtime, but you can read to him
anytime. You can also sing and recite nursery rhymes.
Your baby will get used to the sound of your voice and
find comfort in hearing whatever you have to say.

134. When should I expect to see teeth, and how do I care for them?

The first tooth (usually one of the lower central inci-
sors) typically appears around 6 to 8 months of age,

although some children won't get their first tooth until after 1 year of age. Either way, most kids have all of their baby teeth by age 3 years. Once that first tooth appears, gently wipe it off with a soft washcloth or toothbrush before bed. After 6 months of age, a little fluoride is needed to help prevent cavities. Depending on the concentration of fluoride in your water supply, your pediatrician may recommend simply giving your infant some tap water every day and/or brushing with a tiny bit of fluoride toothpaste at night (a smear of toothpaste the size of a grain of rice) to coat the teeth before bed.

 A note on teething: Teething can be uncomfortable, and your child may drool, put his hands in his mouth, pull or rub his ear, and be a little cranky. These behaviors are normal, and rest assured that they will pass. Teething tablets or gels are not recommended because they are not regulated and may contain chemicals in unknown amounts that may be harmful for your child. See chapter 7, question 72 for more tips on how to handle teething.

Around 1 year of age, gently brush your child's teeth with a tiny bit of fluoride toothpaste twice a day. Make brushing teeth a fun game. Get 3 toothbrushes so your toddler can hold one in each hand, while you brush with the third. Around the age of 1 year or whenever your child gets her first tooth is a good time to see a pediatric dentist. The dentist will let you know if your child needs extra fluoride via water, vitamins, or toothpaste. Follow the dentist's exact recommendation, because too much fluoride can cause permanent white spots on the teeth (this is only cosmetic and not harmful at all, so don't be alarmed if it occurs on your baby's teeth). At about age 2 years, start letting your toddler brush his teeth as well, although you will be doing most of the work. Play a game and take turns. Count to 10 while he attempts to brush, then count to 10 while you brush, and go back and forth a few times. Another idea is to sing a favorite song. A pea-sized amount of fluoride toothpaste can be used at this age. You can start teaching your toddler to rinse and spit, knowing it's going to take a few years to master. It's okay if your child swallows the toothpaste—that's why we use such a small amount! Make sure the toothbrush is the last thing that touches your child's teeth before bedtime. Children typically need some help to ensure good toothbrushing until school age.

If your child's first tooth doesn't appear by 1 year of age or if his teeth look discolored or otherwise abnormal, call your pediatrician for a referral to a pediatric dentist. Early cavities can look like white, yellow, or brown spots and progress to further damage, such as holes or indentations that can be painful and lead to infections.

135.   When does my baby need shoes? Will special shoes help her feet so they don't turn in or out?

Shoes protect your child's feet when she walks on unsafe surfaces or if her feet need to be covered because of weather conditions (rain, sun, or snow). I know those designer shoes you bought are cute, but it's really best to leave your baby barefoot when learning to walk on safe surfaces. Infants learn to walk by gripping the ground with their feet, in a heel-to-toe pattern (which is much easier to do when barefoot). Shoes will not help your child learn to walk sooner, better, or faster. Once you do look for shoes, make sure the shoe is comfortable and flexible and has traction and room for growth. It's best to have a trained professional help find the right fit for your infant or toddler. Young children's feet grow quickly, so they often need to have their shoes checked and refitted every 3 months.

In general, as infants begin to walk, their feet turn slightly outward; over time, they may even turn slightly inward, and with more time they eventually straighten out. Special shoes or braces are typically no longer used for treatment. If you are concerned, let your pediatrician watch your child walk at your next office visit.

136.   At what age can my child learn to swim?

Learning how to swim is a lifesaving skill that is important for everyone. There is evidence that children aged 1 to 4 years may be less likely to drown if they have had formal swim training. If your child enjoys the water (such as taking a bath), can follow instructions, and seems developmentally ready, look for age-appropriate swimming lessons in your area.

In addition to swimming lessons, don't forget the other important layers of protection necessary to keep children safe from drowning. All pools should be surrounded on all 4 sides by a fence (this alone cuts the risk of drowning in half) that is at least 4 feet high and has a self-closing, self-latching gate. With infants, toddlers, and weak swimmers, always use "touch supervision," which means that an adult is always within arm's reach of a child in or near the water. With kids of all ages—even strong swimmers—make sure there is constant supervision by an adult who knows how to swim, perform a rescue, initiate CPR (cardiopulmonary resuscitation), and call for help.

Development

137. Should I be worried that my 4-month-old isn't rolling yet, my 6-month-old isn't sitting alone yet, or my 1-year-old isn't walking yet?

Every child grows and develops at different rates, which is why there is a wide age range for each milestone. In general, if it's only 1 milestone that your infant hasn't hit yet, he may just need a bit more time and encouragement. I've included a chart here to help you know *approximately* what to expect as your child grows.

Your pediatrician will evaluate your child's development at each well-child visit, but if you have any specific concerns or worries, call or schedule an appointment as soon as possible.

Developmental Milestones Chart

Age	Social/ Emotional Milestones	Language Communication Milestones	Cognitive Milestones	Movement/ Physical Development Milestones
2 months	Calms down when spoken to or picked up Looks at your face Seems happy to see you when you walk up to them Smiles when you talk to or smile at them	Makes sounds other than crying Reacts to loud sounds	Watches you as you move Looks at a toy for several seconds	Holds head up when on tummy Moves both arms and both legs Opens hands briefly
4 months	Smiles on their own to get your attention Chuckles (not yet a full laugh) when you try to make them laugh Looks at you, moves, or makes sounds to get or keep your attention	Makes sounds like "ooo," "aahh" Makes sounds back when you talk to them Turns head toward the sound of your voice	If hungry, opens mouth when they see breast or bottle Looks at their hands with interest	Holds head steady without support when you are holding them Holds a toy when you put it in their hands Uses arms to swing at toys Brings hands to mouth Pushes up onto elbows/fore-arms when on tummy

Continued on next page

Age	Social/ Emotional Milestones	Language Communication Milestones	Cognitive Milestones	Movement/ Physical Development Milestones
6 months	Knows familiar people Likes to look at themselves in a mirror Laughs	Takes turns making sounds with you Blows "raspberries" (sticks tongue out and blows) Makes squealing noises	Puts things in mouth to explore them Reaches to grab a toy Closes lips to show they don't want more food	Rolls from tummy to back Pushes up with straight arms when on tummy Leans on hands to support themselves when sitting
9 months	Is shy, clingy, or fearful around strangers Shows several facial expressions, like happy, sad, angry, and surprised Looks when you call their name Reacts when you leave (looks, reaches for you, or cries) Smiles or laughs when you play peek-a-boo	Makes different sounds like 'mamamama' and 'bababababa' Lifts arms up to be picked up	Looks for objects when dropped out of sight (like their spoon or toy) Bangs two things together	Gets to a sitting position by themselves Moves things from one hand to other hand Uses fingers to 'rake' food toward themselves Sits without support
12 months	Plays games with you, like pat-a-cake	Waves 'bye-bye' Calls a parent 'mama' or 'dada' or another special name Understands 'no' (pauses briefly or stops when you say it)	Puts something in a container, like a block in a cup Looks for things they see you hide, like a toy under a blanket	Pulls up to stand Walks, holding onto furniture Drinks from a cup without a lid as you hold it Picks things up between thumb and pointer finger, like small bits of food

Age	Social/ Emotional Milestones	Language Communication Milestones	Cognitive Milestones	Movement/ Physical Development Milestones
18 months	Moves away from you, but looks to make sure you are close by Points to show you something interesting Puts hands out for you to wash them Looks at a few pages in a book with you Helps you dress them by pushing arm through sleeve or lifting up foot	Tries to say three or more words besides "mama" or "dada" Follows one-step directions without any gestures, like giving you the toy when you say, "Give it to me."	Copies you doing chores, like sweeping with a broom Plays with toys in a simple way, like pushing a toy car	Walks without holding onto anyone or anything Scribbles Drinks from a cup without a lid and may spill sometimes Feeds themselves their fingers Tries to use a spoon Climbs on and off a couch or chair without help
2 years	Notices when others are hurt or upset, like pausing or looking sad when someone is crying Looks at your face to see how to react in a new situation	Points to things in a book when you ask, like "Where is the bear?" Says at least two words together, like "More milk." Points to at least two body parts when you ask them to show you Uses more gestures than just waving and pointing, like blowing a kiss or nodding yes	Holds something in one hand while using the other hand; for example, holding a container and taking the lid off Tries to use switches, knobs, or buttons on a toy Plays with more than one toy at the same time, like putting toy food on a toy plate	Kicks a ball Runs Walks (not climbs) up a few stairs with or without help Eats with a spoon

Continued on next page

Age	Social/ Emotional Milestones	Language Communication Milestones	Cognitive Milestones	Movement/ Physical Development Milestones
30 months	Plays next to other children and sometimes plays with them Shows you what they can do by saying, "Look at me!" Follows simple routines when told, like helping to pick up toys when you say, "It's clean-up time."	Says about 50 words Says two or more words, with one action word, like "Doggie run" Names things in a book when you point and ask, "What is this?" Says words like "I," "me," or "we"	Uses things to pretend, like feeding a block to a doll as if it were food Shows simple problem-solving skills, like standing on a small stool to reach something Follows two-step instructions like "Put the toy down and close the door." Shows they know at least one color, like pointing to a red crayon when you ask, "Which one is red?"	Uses hands to twist things, like turning doorknobs or unscrewing lids Takes some clothes off by themselves, like loose pants or an open jacket Jumps off the ground with both feet Turns book pages, one at a time, when you read to them

Age	Social/ Emotional Milestones	Language Communication Milestones	Cognitive Milestones	Movement/ Physical Development Milestones
3 years	Calms down within 10 minutes after you leave them, like at a child care drop-off Notices other children and joins them to play	Talks with you in conversation using at least two back-and-forth exchanges Asks "who," "what," "where," or "why" questions, like "Where is mommy/daddy?" Says what action is happening in a picture or book when asked, like "running," "eating," or "playing" Says first name, when asked Talks well enough for others to understand most of the time	Draws a circle when you show them how Avoids touching hot objects, like a stove, when you warn them	Strings items together, like large beads or macaroni Puts on some clothes by themselves, like loose pants or a jacket Uses a fork

138.   My 3-year-old is stuttering. Should I worry?

Toddlers and preschoolers may often repeat sounds, syllables, or words when they speak. Many times, these speech errors (also known as *dysfluencies*) are part of normal development and may come and go as children rapidly acquire new vocabulary. Such speech errors usually occur at the beginning of a sentence when a child is formulating her thought. Most children this age will outgrow these dysfluencies without any intervention. Children with such normal types of stuttering typically appear unaware of the extra sounds they are making and show little frustration.

Strategies to assist your child include slowing down your speech (if you are a fast talker), asking one question at a time, and being patient. It is important to give your child time to speak, without correcting him.

If your child is repeating syllables 4 or more times (such as d-d-d-d-dog instead of d-d-dog) or if your child is prolonging a sound (such as ddddddddog), this is more concerning.

In addition, you should ask your pediatrician for a referral to a speech therapist if you observe the following:

- ☐ Your child's facial muscles appear to be tense during speaking.
- ☐ Your child seems uncomfortable or stressed getting the words out.
- ☐ There are other unusual facial movements or blinking (in such cases additional specialists may also be needed).

139.   What are the signs of autism?

Autism spectrum disorder is a complex developmental disorder, with a spectrum of symptoms that range
from mild to severe. It is more common in boys,
and although signs can be found as early as infancy,
autism is typically noticed between 18 months and
3 years of age. Your pediatrician should screen for
autism at the 18- and 24-month checkups, as well as
survey your child's development at every well-child
visit. Diagnosis as early as possible is important
because research has shown that early intervention
programs can improve the outcomes for a child with
autism spectrum disorder. It is also important to note
that there are other developmental issues that may
cause symptoms similar to those of autism. As always,
talk to your pediatrician if you have any concerns
about your child's development.

Here are some common signs of autism:

- ☐ Delayed or absent speech
- ☐ Lack of eye contact and response when calling
  your child's name
- ☐ Shows little or no response to your smile or other
  facial expressions
- ☐ Lack of gestures, such as pointing
- ☐ Does not look at an object you point at
- ☐ Does not bring and show you favorite objects
  or items
- ☐ Doesn't like hugs and kisses

- ☐ Repetitive behavior (such as lining up toys in same order) or words (aka echoing)
- ☐ Plays with parts of toy instead of entire toy (eg, spinning wheels on toy car)
- ☐ Difficult behavior
- ☐ Delayed milestones, especially language and social skills
- ☐ Unusual reactions to the way things look, feel, smell, taste, or sound

 If you think your child may have autism spectrum disorder, talk to your pediatrician. Early intensive therapy (eg, speech therapy, occupational therapy, behavioral therapy, social integration) can lessen these symptoms and bring about a substantial improvement.

140. What are the signs of attention-deficit/hyperactivity disorder (ADHD)?

Attention-deficit/hyperactivity disorder can cause a child to have difficulty paying attention, hyperactivity, and/or impulsive behaviors. It is a developmental disorder that is not typically diagnosed in infants and toddlers but is observed more often in children 4 to 18 years old, after they have started attending school. The reason for this is that some of the symptoms of ADHD are considered "normal" in toddlers, such as not paying attention, having trouble sitting still, and continuously running around. It really isn't until such behaviors begin interfering with school and other activities that a diagnosis is assigned.

These behaviors become more apparent once a child enters school because there are more rules to adhere to and more group activities that require concentration and self-control. Children with ADHD also may have trouble learning in school. If your child is already in preschool, speak with her teacher about your concerns and ask if the teacher has noticed any of the same behaviors. Often, teachers are the first ones to bring ADHD concerns to parents. Some behaviors may be normal for a child's age, while others may warrant further attention and/or assessment (not all children who have difficulty concentrating or hyperactive behavior have ADHD).

 Talk to your pediatrician if you notice any concerning behaviors in your child. She can evaluate and test your child for ADHD or refer you to a specialist. Behavioral therapy, where you as a parent may have the opportunity to participate, is often the first step in treating ADHD. In addition, proper nutrition that includes supplements such as omega-3 fatty acids, proper sleep, exercise, and screen-free time can help. Later on, medication may be necessary. Most children respond well to therapy and/or medication and are able to keep their symptoms under good control and be successful, productive children, teens, and adults.

Turn Off the Television!

The American Academy of Pediatrics recommends that children younger than 18 months not be exposed to television, videos, or video or computer games (this includes phones and tablets). The first 2 years are especially important in the growth and development of your child's brain. During this time, children need good, positive interaction with other children and adults and hands-on exploration to develop properly. Too much television can negatively affect early brain development.

After age 18 months to 2 years, limit your child to no more than 1 hour a day of educational, nonviolent screen time. Make sure programs are age appropriate, and always watch or play video games or apps with your child so that you know the content she's being exposed to and can discuss it with her. This is a perfect opportunity to teach your child life lessons and bring up important topics, such as health and safety.

Not all screens (television, computers, phones, tablets) are bad. In fact, you can use them to your advantage if you choose educational programs to watch for a limited amount of time each day and discuss them with your child. Some examples of high-quality programming for children include *PBS Kids* and *Sesame Street.* In addition, video chatting has become a useful tool for communicating with family members and friends remotely. I know my boys as toddlers looked forward to "FaceTiming with Grammie." This kind of media use is fine in moderation and can help maintain important family or social connections.

It's always a good idea to avoid using screens during meal-times and 1 hour before bedtime, as they can disrupt family bonding and sleep and lead to bad habits later on. Try to avoid using a screen as a distraction to calm your child down (of course, there are some rare situations in which this may be all right, including watching a screen during a painful medical procedure or other severely stressful event). As long as the screen time provides a positive and useful source of interaction with your child, it becomes a tool rather than a mindless distraction. Ask your pediatrician if you have questions about the media your child is watching or using. She may have some more recommendations about media use that are specific to your child and family. Commonsensemedia.org is a great resource to find age-appropriate programs, apps, and games for your child.

Behavior

141. What is the best way to deal with temper tantrums?

The key to discipline is consistency. Remember, *you* are the parent. Temper tantrums can be challenging to deal with, but they can also be minimized. Most of the time, children are looking for attention (whether positive attention via praise or negative attention that results in punishment or scolding). The idea is to encourage good behavior by providing positive reinforcement, ignore bad behavior when possible (as long as there is no immediate danger), and set firm limits or consequences for completely unacceptable behaviors. Here are some tips you can use to help stop (or at least decrease) the tantrums.

☐ Ignore the behavior. If you walk away or don't pay attention, your child will likely stop.

☐ Put your child in time-out. Pick a location in your house where your child must sit or stand for a few minutes (1 minute per year of age) or until she calms down.

☐ Refocus your child on something else. I like to walk to the other side of the room, announce that "mommy is going to read a book," and start reading out loud. My sons would usually quiet down and come join me.

☐ Give your child a task to complete so that she feels helpful and involved (this works well if you have multiple children and one of them is feeling left out).

☐ Provide praise when your child is behaving nicely. Catch her doing something good and reward her. Make sure to specify the action or behavior you are praising to promote more of these good behaviors in the future.

☐ Empower your child and help her have a little control by offering her small, simple choices to make during your daily routine versus "yes" or "no" answers. For example, do you want to put your shirt or your pants on first? Or would you like to eat an apple or a banana for your snack this afternoon?

☐ Avoid situations that are likely to bring on a tantrum. If your child always melts down on your second errand, then limit each outing to one errand at a time. If your child is more likely to have a tantrum when hungry, pack a healthy snack or two in your bag for such situations.

☐ Leave the location. If you are in a public place (eg, grocery store, restaurant), simply take your child and leave if she throws a tantrum. It's hard to do when you're in the checkout line or in the middle of a meal, but it will calm her down and teach her that when she behaves like that, the activity will stop.

Thumb-sucking

Thumb-sucking is a common self-soothing behavior that usually begins in the first year. It isn't dangerous, and toddlers eventually outgrow it—typically by the time they start kindergarten. You can't take the thumb away, but you can try introducing another "lovey" or comfort item, such as a special toy or blanky that your child can carry around. Applying adhesive strips, splints, or yucky-tasting solutions to your child's thumb isn't very effective in the first few years. The best method of action is to ignore the behavior, take comfort in the fact that your toddler has a quiet method of soothing herself, and wait it out. If it becomes a major problem, ask your pediatrician about a technique called *habit reversal training*.

Dr. Tanya's Tip

Changing Behavior—It Takes a Week

Almost any behavior can be modified within 1 week, as long as all caregivers are consistent and provide encouragement and praise. Whether you're trying to stop your toddler from biting or getting him to sleep all night in a big-boy bed, 1 week is usually all you need, as long as you stick with it (you can do it!). Here are some tips for changing your child's behavior.

Be consistent—have all caregivers keep the same rules and routine.

Encourage—read an encouraging book on the topic or tell a story.

Have rewards—praise him for doing well; offer hugs and kisses, stickers, or a small token.

Anticipate conflict—change your routine to avoid battle situations.

Very quick response—immediately follow your child's action with a consequence (good or bad).

Ignore—minor, undesirable actions often aren't worth your energy.

One at a time—pick your battle and choose only one behavior to modify at a time.

Role model—your child watches you and follows your lead, so demonstrate good behavior, respect, and love for those around you.

Potty Training

142. When can I toilet train my child, and how do I do it?

Many children are ready to start potty training when they are around 2½ years old, so at your child's 2-year checkup, ask your pediatrician when to start. Once you get the go-ahead, the first thing to do is take a deep breath and relax. Everyone eventually learns how to use the potty. If your child isn't ready or if you're feeling pressured by a preschool start date or the birth of a sibling, inevitably the potty training won't happen and may even take longer. If you wait until your toddler is truly ready, it's much easier on everyone involved. In case you're wondering, the age at which your toddler eventually learns how to use the toilet has no bearing on how smart he is or his future academic success. No college application or future employer is going to ask him at what age he learned to use the potty. Signs that your toddler may be ready include the following:

- ☐ He stays dry for several hours at a time.
- ☐ He has regular, predictable bowel movements.
- ☐ He shows signs he is about to go in his diaper, such as hiding or squatting.
- ☐ He seems uncomfortable when his diaper is dirty and asks to be changed.
- ☐ He follows simple instructions, walks to the bathroom, and helps undress himself.

☐ He asks to use the toilet and wear big-kid underwear.

To be truly toilet trained, your toddler has to be able to sense that he needs to go, be able to interpret that sensation, and then be able to tell you and take some action (actually get the pee or poop into the potty). Typically, this happens around 2½ years of age, but it can be earlier or later.

Prepping for toilet training can actually begin earlier. Here are some steps you can take to achieve success.

Start "potty talk": Teach your child the words that your family will use for potty-related things, like *toilet, stool,* and *urine.* (*Potty, poop,* and *pee* seem to be very acceptable these days, but be careful. Whatever words you use, your child will repeat in public—possibly while grocery shopping.) Tell your child what he just did in the potty or the action you are taking, such as, "Jacob just went poop!" or "Let's change your dirty diaper." Kids are smart. He will catch on quickly and start telling you when he goes or that he needs to be changed.

Check for soft stools: Make sure your child's stools are soft. If he is constipated and his stool is hard, he won't want to go in the potty because pooping hurts. He'll hold onto his stool, making it larger, harder, and more painful, and potty training will not be successful. (For stool-softening tips, see question 55, on page 98.)

See one, do one: Make a point of announcing when you need to go to the bathroom, and let your child watch you use the toilet. Teach him to always wash his hands afterward.

Decide on a big or a little potty: It's up to you if you want to buy a smaller potty chair for your child (let him help pick it out or write his name on it!) or just place a stool or toilet seat insert (choose something cute, like a favorite character, that will excite him) for him to use. Either way, it helps if he has something to push his feet against. Have you ever tried to poop with your feet off the ground? It's not easy.

Create fun and games: Make potty time fun for him— read a story while he's sitting on the potty, or pass the time by singing a song. There are several good books about using the potty that will encourage him to do it. Try not to scold him for not going or force him to sit there if he can't go. It works much better if you praise his efforts, however small they are. Reward your child with positive words, big hugs, kisses, or a special potty song or dance. If needed, you can always offer him a sticker, stamp, or small treat if he uses the potty, as well.

Emphasize handwashing: Make it easy for your child to get to all the tools he needs to wash his hands. Place a small step stool in the bathroom for him to be able to reach the sink (even if you are helping him up). Keep the soap and towels within reach, as well. Have fun and teach your child to sing a short song like "Happy Birthday" while washing to ensure that he scrubs his hands for enough time.

Dry at Night

Potty training refers to daytime use of the toilet. Nighttime dryness for most kids doesn't happen until much later. In fact, it's perfectly normal for kids to still urinate at night up until 6 years of age, and sometimes even longer. So put your child in absorbent training pants, disposable training pants, or a diaper at night (you can call it "nighttime underwear") until your child is dry most nights. Make going to the bathroom part of your child's bedtime routine to increase the chances of having success with staying dry at night. Don't scold your child for bed-wetting—accidents will happen. Talk to your pediatrician if you have concerns about your child and bed-wetting.

143. My 3-year-old knows how to use the toilet, but she will only use it sometimes. I'm tired of alternating between underwear and training pants. What should I do?

If your child has had some success with potty training and knows what to do, then choosing not to use the potty may be a behavioral issue. It can be confusing for her to sometimes wear big-girl underwear and other times wear diapers or pull-ups. Choose a long weekend when you can be home with her the entire time, and let her know the day before that starting tomorrow, she gets to wear big-girl underwear all the time. Then, buy a big stack of underwear, get rid of all the diapers and pull-ups, and go for it! Use a reward system, such as placing a stamp on her hand or a phone call to Grandma or Grandpa every time she goes in the potty. If she has an accident, acknowledge it ("Oops, you had an accident"), have her help clean up ("Let's dump the poop in the potty and rinse your clothes in the sink"), and move on ("Next time, let Mommy know and I'll help you get to the potty in time"). If you are consistent and don't go backwards (resist the urge to put her in diapers for car rides or trips to the store), your child will probably be potty trained in less than a week. Remember to not get discouraged. Potty training can be difficult, but keep up the good work, and you and your child will soon see the results!

CHAPTER 14

Sleep

Sleep is by far the most popular topic of the parenting workshops I conduct in my practice, and it's definitely one of the most important. Who doesn't want a few more z's every night? The reality is that in the first few weeks at home with your newborn, you probably won't get much sleep, and the first few months can be hit or miss. But after that, if you play your cards right, you and your baby can start sleeping well—at least most of the time. So, how do you stack the odds in your favor? A bedtime routine, consistency, and a little willpower can make all the difference. That said, even the best-laid plans at 6 pm won't always go according to schedule when it's 4 am, you're sleep deprived, and you're having to make quick decisions. But stay on track and keep your goal in mind—to sleep all night long!

While I have found success with the following techniques, your pediatrician can help make adjustments as needed for your child.

Sleep Solutions

144. I'm so exhausted. When will my baby sleep through the night, and how can I make that happen?

I hear you. Having been through it myself 3 times, I can tell you that my only solace at the time was knowing that my sons' sleep schedules would improve and that, by around 4 to 6 months of age, they would hopefully be sleeping 8 hours a night. So, here's the plan.

First 2 months after birth: During this time, your baby still needs to feed when he wakes up every 3 to 4 hours. Start a regular bedtime routine so he can learn that this is nighttime and not nap time. The routine doesn't need to be long. It may work well to include a bath, pajamas, book, feeding, swaddle, getting put to bed, and having lights out. Your baby will probably fall asleep during the feeding, or you can rock him to sleep, which is fine for now.

Three to 4 months: Continue the bedtime routine, but end with placing your baby in his crib awake, so he can learn how to put himself to sleep. If feeding always puts him to sleep, reverse your routine so you feed him first, end with pajamas or story time, and put him to bed when he's awake.

If he gets used to being rocked or fed to sleep, he will need you to perform these rituals when he wakes up in the middle of the night. When he does wake up at night, give him a few minutes before you jump in and feed him. Often it's just a wakeful part of his sleep cycle, and he'll drift off again on his own.

Four to 6 months: Your baby most likely does not need to feed anymore in the middle of the night, so he should be able to sleep for 6 to 8 hours (if you let him). Keep your bedtime routine consistent and allow him to fall asleep on his own. When he wakes up in the middle of the night, allow him to use the same self-soothing skills to put himself back to sleep. As you wean your baby from the nighttime feeding, he may cry a bit (or a lot) as he learns how to put himself back to sleep. Give him time to do this. Within a few nights, he will figure out how to soothe himself back to sleep. Developing good sleep habits is important (for everyone in the house!).

After 6 months: Your baby should be able to sleep at least 8 hours straight at night. If not, this is a good time to improve your bedtime routine and nighttime sleep plan (see question 147, on page 257).

Sudden Infant Death Syndrome

Sudden infant death syndrome (SIDS) is the unexplained death of a child younger than 1 year. The exact cause is unknown. To decrease your baby's risk of SIDS, always put him to sleep on his back, don't share a bed with your baby, don't expose your baby to cigarette smoke, and use a firm mattress without pillows, blankets, bumper pads, toys, or extra-soft bedding. Sleep sacks and wearable blankets are good options to keep your baby warm while sleeping. The American Academy of Pediatrics now recommends that infants should sleep in their parents' room until they are 6 to 12 months old, without sharing the same bed. It has been found that room sharing decreases the risk of SIDS by up to 50%! So, be sure to tell grandparents and other care-givers of these recommendations if they will be putting your child to sleep.

145. Do you recommend using apnea monitors or new fancy tech gadgets that monitor a baby's breathing and heart rate to prevent SIDS?

Generally speaking, no. Unless you have a premature baby who leaves the neonatal intensive care unit with an apnea monitor or your pediatrician prescribes one for another reason, such devices are not routinely rec-ommended for babies, and they have not been shown to decrease the risk of SIDS. Some parents may buy a device to monitor their baby while sleeping anyway, for peace of mind, or because it's the latest baby gadget on the market. But getting frequent false alarms may be more disruptive to sleep (and mental health) than helpful. Your best bet is to save your money and forego the fancy monitor, keep your baby in your room at night, and follow the safe sleep recommendations of the American Academy of Pediatrics (which appear here, in the Sudden Infant Death Syndrome text box).

146. My son sleeps so much less than my daughter did at this age. How do I know he is getting enough sleep?

Sleep is important for your child's brain development and growth. Lack of sleep can contribute to irritability, inattention, hyperactivity, and other unpleasant childhood behaviors. Getting enough sleep can help your child with learning, emotional regulation, and overall quality of life. Every child needs sleep (parents do too!), but how many hours of sleep are needed depends on the child. For children younger than 4 months of age, the amount of sleep needed varies widely. After 4 months of age, your child requires sleep in the following ranges:

☐ Infants 4–12 months of age: 12 to 16 hours (including naps)

- ☐ Toddlers 1–2 years old: 11 to 14 hours
  (including naps)
- ☐ Children 3–5 years old: 10 to 13 hours
  (including naps)
- ☐ Children 6–12 years old: 9 to 12 hours
- ☐ If your child seems cranky during the day,
  though, getting an extra hour of sleep is usually
  a good idea.

Improve Your Child's Quality of Sleep

Here are some tips to help improve your child's quality of
sleep (and your sanity).

Before Bed

- ☐ Make sure your child is active during the day. This will
  help him fall asleep faster at night.
- ☐ Avoid stimulating activities an hour before bed (such as
  television, tablets, and video games).

Sleep Environment

- ☐ Avoid having TV, tablets, phones, and other electronics
  in your child's bedroom.
- ☐ Keep the bedroom cool, dark, and quiet.
- ☐ Try to limit disruptive circumstances (such as a bedroom facing a loud street or a shared bedroom with an
  older child who has a later bedtime).

Bedtime Routines

☐ Consistency is key. Stick to the same time, place, and sequence of bedtime events as much as possible.

☐ Many families swear by the "4 B's": Breast/Bottle, Bath, Book, Bed.

 If you think your child isn't getting enough sleep despite your best attempts, talk to your child's pediatrician. In some cases, an underlying sleep disorder may be the cause of poor sleep, and specific treatment may be needed.

---

147. My infant/toddler wakes up in the middle of the night and screams until I nurse her, rock her, bring her into my bed, or give her a pacifier. I can't bear to hear her cry. How can I get her to sleep through the night?

How you respond to your child in the middle of the night can either extinguish or encourage the unwanted behavior.

After 4 to 6 months of age, if you always nurse, rock, cuddle, or "pacify" your baby in the middle of the night, she will become accustomed to needing your help to fall back asleep. Nighttime is sleep time, and unless you want to continue doing this for the next year or longer, give your child the chance to learn how to put herself back to sleep. It's much easier now than when she's standing up in her crib, yelling for mommy. Yes, she may scream and cry. I know it's hard for you to hear. I know you may worry, but you have all day to cuddle with her, show her how much you love her, and let her know you're there for her. Also, since you're probably wondering if she needs to be fed in the middle of the night, she usually doesn't. Waking up wanting to be fed is often just a habit. From 4 to 6 months of age, most babies should easily be able to go 6 to 8 hours at night without food, and after 6 months of age, most babies can go at least 8 to 10 hours. Once you stop feeding your child in the middle of the night, she'll make up for it by eating more during the day.

After 6 to 8 months of age, the best approach is to let your child figure out how to put herself back to sleep in the middle of the night. Pick a night to begin letting her self-soothe. A Friday night often works well, because the first few nights of not comforting her in the night might be tough. Be consistent, because she won't understand why you pick her up and feed her sometimes, but other times you don't. Let her fall asleep at bedtime, and tell her how long you expect her to sleep (saying it out loud helps you know your plan). Then, when she does wake up, allow her to figure out how to get back to sleep on her own. There may be a few nights of crying, but if you resist the temptation to intervene, the crying will be less each night, and before you know it, she'll be sleeping all night long (and so will you). In the morning, tell her how proud you are of her—clap, cheer, sing, or dance. Even if she is too young to understand, it's a good routine to start. Also, both parents must be on the same page for any sleep plan to work, so talk to your partner and agree on a consistent approach.

Toddler Troubles

148. My toddler wakes up at night, gets out of his bed, and comes into our room. If I try to put him back in bed, he throws a fit and wakes up his siblings or the neighbors. What can I do?

For those of you whose child is still sleeping in a crib, I'm telling you now—it's much easier and safer to sleep-train a toddler in a crib, before he can get out of bed and roam around the house. No matter what the age, it's hard to let a child cry when you know it will disturb other people. Before starting sleep training, warn everyone who will be able to hear your child crying (buy the neighbors a present), and then spend a few consecutive nights resolving the problem. Once your child is sleeping through the night, everyone will benefit.

Much like the previous question, how you respond to your child in the middle of the night can either extinguish or encourage the unwanted behavior. Again, set aside a few nights in a row where it's okay if you don't get any sleep (maybe a long weekend). Keep your bedtime routine consistent. Let your child know what's expected of him—to sleep all night long in his own bed. Give him a special new pillow, blanky, or stuffed animal that he can cuddle with in the middle of the night. Let him know it is there to help him sleep all night in his own big-kid bed.

When your child does get out of bed, take his hand and march him back to bed. Simply say, "At night, we sleep in our own bed." Tuck him in and leave. The next time he gets out, say "bed." Take his hand and escort him back to bed. The third time, don't say anything. Just take him back to bed. Continue this routine every time he gets out of bed. The next night, do the same thing. It should only take 3 or 4 nights in a row (allow an entire week, just in case) before you are all sleeping through the night in your own beds. You may want to put a safety gate at your child's door so you can leave the door open to hear him, but the gate will keep him from getting out and roaming around the house at night alone. In the morning, tell him how proud you are of him— dance, cheer, throw a party, or do whatever it takes to encourage everyone in the house to continue the routine.

Dr. Tanya's Tip

From Crib to Big-Kid Bed

Once your child is tall enough to climb out of the crib (at least 3 feet tall), she should start sleeping in a big-kid bed. Make sure the bed is placed a safe distance away from dressers or other items that she could climb or roll onto and injure herself. Continue your bedtime routine, but end it by reminding her that she must stay in bed until you come to get her in the morning.

Here are some steps to help your child transition to a big-kid bed.

Build excitement—find a book (or make up a story) on the topic to get your toddler ready. Include her when choosing bedding for her new big bed.

Introduce a "lovey"—explain that a special blanky, stuffed animal, or doll can sleep in her big bed too.

Go for it—pick a night to have her start sleeping in the bed, and don't go back to using a crib.

Bedtime routine—keep your previous bedtime routine and be consistent.

Encourage good sleep habits—praise and reward her (hugs and kisses work well) at bedtime and every morning when she has stayed in her big-kid bed all night.

Don't forget safety—install a bed rail or remove the bed from the frame so the mattress is low to the ground. Keep her room safe in case she gets out of bed. Consider using a door gate for her bedroom to keep her from wandering around the house at night.

149. My toddler wakes up at night and screams. Is she having nightmares? Or are these the night terrors I've heard about?

While both nightmares and night terrors can be scary for parents and interrupt everyone's sleep, the 2 are very different.

Night terrors usually occur in children older than 18 months—usually in the first third of the night. The typical scenario is that a child wakes up approximately 3 hours after going to sleep, acting like she is possessed. She may scream, shake, and point at things. She may have a confused or glassy-eyed look and cry uncontrollably. This can be terrifying to witness. The child cannot be comforted (she may even try to push you away if you try to hold her) and doesn't even know you're in the room. But she easily goes back to sleep after the episode. The next morning, the child doesn't remember the event, although everyone else in the house will. While most night terror episodes last for 10 minutes or less, they can last as long as 45 minutes.

Stress and tiredness can contribute to night terrors, so evaluate and make changes if possible to help your child's schedule and routine. Try to put her to bed a little earlier at night or make sure she gets a nap if she still needs one. What can you do to break the cycle? Because night terrors generally occur around the same time every night, wake your child up about 15 to 30 minutes prior to the expected episode every night for a

week, and then let her fall back to sleep. This will interrupt her sleep cycle, and her body will jump into the
next stage of sleep, when the terrors don't occur.

Nightmares typically happen during the second
half of the night. Kids with nightmares will wake up
fully and respond to parental comforting. They may
remember the dream, even the next day. Providing
reassurance each time your child has a nightmare can
help prevent the nightmare from happening again.
Talk to your child about the dreams and explain that
they are not real. Take a look at your child's environment (eg, preschool, home) and determine if anything
is bothering her. Be sure to avoid exposing your child
to violent activity, movies, or television shows. Try
keeping a nightlight and a special dream catcher in
her room if they make her feel better. Talk to your
pediatrician if the nightmares persist for more than a
few days.

150. My child snores. What does this mean?

Many children snore on and off, and up to 10% of
children snore on a regular basis. Occasional snoring can be caused by allergies or colds and is usually
not worrisome. Regular nighttime snoring, especially
when associated with gasps, snorts, or intermittent
pauses, can be a sign of a more serious condition
called *obstructive sleep apnea*. Children with obstructive sleep apnea sometimes have daytime sleepiness
or more commonly behavioral problems because they

aren't getting quality sleep or enough oxygen at night. Sometimes, it is caused by overly large tonsils and adenoids, which may be worse if your child is overweight. If your child snores regularly, discuss it with your pediatrician. He may recommend a sleep study (a study in which your child is observed while sleeping, and her breathing and heart rate are measured) to rule out sleep apnea and/or refer you to an ear, nose, and throat doctor for evaluation.

Index

A

AAP. *See* American Academy of Pediatrics (AAP)
ABO incompatibility, 171
Abscesses, skin, 138
Acetaminophen (Tylenol)
    after vaccines, 160
    for air travel, 13
    as diaper bag essential, 9
    dosing chart, 126
    for fever, 126
    for hand, foot, and mouth
        disease, 146
    for insect bite or sting, 222
    for pain after falling, 211
    for sore throat or mouth
        pain, 145
    taken while breastfeeding, 55
    for teething, 130
Acne, baby, 176
Additives in infant formula,
    59–60
Adenoids, 264
Adenovirus, 146
ADHD. *See* Attention-deficit/
    hyperactivity disorder
    (ADHD)

Advil. *See* Ibuprofen (Motrin
    or Advil)
Air travel, 12–13
Alcohol, 6, 54–55
Allergies
    bottle-feeding, 58–59, 67
    breastfeeding, 52
    eczema due to, 67, 78, 149,
        184–185
    life-threatening, 187
    milk and other liquids, 79,
        80, 88–89
    solid food. *See* Food
        allergies
    when to call pediatrician
        about, 187
Almond butter, 80
Almond milk, 90
Aluminum salts, 162–163
American Academy of
    Pediatrics (AAP)
    breastfeeding, 36
    infant vitamins, 38
    *New Mother's Guide to
        Breastfeeding,* 32
    pacifiers, 18
    rear-facing car seats, 218

American Academy of
     Pediatrics (AAP)
     (*continued*)
  room sharing with baby, 5,
     254
  television, videos, and video
     or computer games,
     240–241
  toddler vitamins, 81
  vaccines, 166
  vitamin K injection after
     birth, 4
  when to introduce solid
     foods, 75
Amino acid–based formulas, 88
Anaphylaxis, 78
Angel kiss, 189–190
Animal bites, 222–223
Antibiotics, 137–138
  for ear infections, 142
  eye medication, 141
  green mucus and need for,
     148
  loose stools after, 105–106
  for methicillin-resistant
     Staphylococcus aureus
     (MRSA), 180–181
  for scarlet fever, 147
  topical, 179, 223
Antifungal cream, 175
Antihistamines, 55, 187, 222
Antimicrobial soap, 181
Apnea monitors, 254–255
Appendicitis, 111–112
Applesauce, 103
Apricots, 100
ARA. *See* Arachidonic acid
     (ARA)
Arachidonic acid (ARA), 57, 60

Aspirin, 126
Asthma, 149
  nighttime coughing with, 156
Atopic dermatitis. *See* Eczema
Attention-deficit/hyperactiv-
     ity disorder (ADHD),
     238–239
Au pairs, 196
Autism
  signs of, 237–238
  vaccines and, 161–162
Avocados, 75, 77, 78

B

Baby bag, 9–10
Baby blues and mood swings,
     6–7
Baby carriers/slings, 5
Babyproofing, 219–220
Baby wipes, 9, 174
Bacterial infections
  fever due to, 120
  methicillin-resistant
     Staphylococcus aureus
     (MRSA), 180–181
Bananas, 78, 103
Barley, 45
Bassinets, 5
Bathing
  after circumcision, 28
  baby acne, 176
  bleach and, 181
  ear infections and, 144–145
  eczema and, 184–185
  sponge, for fever, 129
  umbilical cord stump, 21–22
  for uncircumcised baby,
     28–29
Beans, 53

Bed-wetting, 248
Behavior modification, 244
Belly button, 20–22
Bicycling legs, 14
Bifidobacterium probiotics, 33, 39, 60
"Big Eight" foods, 79–81
Big-kid beds, 261
Bilirubin, 170–173
Birthmarks, 189–191
Bisphenol A (BPA), 62–63
Bites
    animal, 222–223
    insect, 221–222
Blanket sleepers, 17
Blankets/nursing covers, 9
    as comfort items, 243
    for swaddling, 15–17
Bleach, 181
Blessed thistle, 45
Blood type, 171
Body parts, 20–22
Body temperature, baby's, 12
Bonding
    baby carrier/sling for, 5
    in the delivery room, 3
    skin-to-skin contact for, 3, 5
    through bottle-feeding, 4–5
    through breastfeeding, 4
Bottle-feeding, 57–68
    allergies to cow's milk protein and, 58–59, 67
    baby bottle tooth decay due to, 68
    boiling water for, 64
    bonding through, 4
    deciding between breastfeeding and, 57
    ear infections and, 142

European/Australian formula standards for, 61
formula additives for, 59–60
formula preparations for, 60–61
gas with, 66–67
infant formula as healthy for, 57
main types of formulas for, 58–59
nipples for, 63–64
premixing powder formula for, 62
pumped breast milk for, 40–43
supplies for, 9
switching of formulas for, 59, 66–67
transition to sippy cups from, 84–86
types of bottles for, 62–63
warming formula for, 64–65
Botulism, 81, 156
BPA. *See* Bisphenol A (BPA)
Bread, 99, 103
Breast cream, 46
Breast engorgement, 48
Breastfeeding, 31–55
    alcohol and caffeine consumption while, 54–55
    baby falling asleep while, 44
    baby spitting up when, 52–53
    benefits of, 33
    bonding through, 4
    breaking the latch, 49
    breast engorgement and, 48
    child care and, 200
    comfortable positioning for, 50–51

Breastfeeding (*continued*)
  creating a nursing station
    for, 42
  deciding between formula
    and, 57
  ear infections and, 33, 143
  feeding on demand, 37–38
  first attempt at, 3
  help and information on,
    31–32
  hunger cues and, 37
  jaundice, 171–172
  lactation consultants for,
    32, 46, 57
  New Mother's Guide to
    Breastfeeding book on,
    32
  pacifier interference with, 18
  preterm infants, 34–35
  proper positioning for
    latch, 48–49
  pumping for. *See* Pumping,
    breast milk
  schedule for, 37–38
  sore nipples and, 46–47
  of twins, 37
  vitamin supplementation
    for, 38–39
  while having a cold, 53–54
Breast milk
  antibodies passed through, 53
  benefits of, 33
  colostrum, 35
  coming in, 35–36
  donor, 34
  engorgement and, 48
  pumping of, 40–41
  for removing mucus from
    nose, 23
  storage of, 41–42
  tips to increase supply of,
    45
Breast milk cookies, 45
Breast pumps, 41
Breathing
  food allergy and trouble, 78
  nasal congestion and, 23–25
  retractions, 24, 152, 153
  signs of troubled, 24–25
  transitional, 35–36
  wheezing, 148–149
Breathing treatments, 151
Broccoli, 53, 83, 89, 99
Bronchiolitis, 149, 150
  treatment for, 151–152
Bronchodilators, 149
Brown rice, 76
Burp cloths/washcloths, 9, 52,
  73
Burping, 72

C

Cabbage, 89
Caffeine, 6
Calamine lotion, 222
Calcium, 6, 91
Candida albicans, 175
Cantharidin, 182
Carrots
  pureed, 75
  raw, 81
Car seats, 216–218
  flat head and, 26
Cauliflower, 53, 99
Cavities, 228
CDC. *See* Centers for Disease
  Control and Prevention
  (CDC)

Centers for Disease Control and Prevention (CDC)
   breast milk storage, 42
   vaccines, 166
Cephalohematoma, 171
Cereals
   for diarrhea, 103
   fortified, 76–77, 89
   white rice, 76–77
   whole-grain, 77, 80, 99
Cetirizine, 222
Chamomile tea, 110
Changing pad, 9
Cheese, 91
Cherries, 100
Chest pain, 153
Chicken, 76, 77
Chickenpox, 159, 168
Childbirth, 2–3
   baby blues after, 6–7
Child care, 193–203
   for after delivery, 193–194
   breastfeeding and, 200
   differences between in-home and facility, 197–198
   in home, 195–198
   illness exposures in, 201
   preschools, 202–203
   sick policies for, 197–198, 200–201
   "what if" questions to ask about, 199
   when to begin and what to look for, 194–195
Children, amount of sleep needed by, 255–256
Choking hazards, 81, 208
Circumcision

bleeding and infection after, 30
   calling the pediatrician about, 28
   dark yellow or bloody stain on diaper, 28
   Gomco, Sheldon, or Mogen clamp, 27–28
   medical benefits of, 27
   penis sticking to diaper, 28
   Plastibell, 27
Citrus foods, 52
Clothing, baby, 9, 11–12
   removed for fever, 129
   for sun protection, 183
Cluster feeding, 37
Cognitive milestones, 231–235
Coins, ingestion of, 207–208
Colds. See Coughs, colds, and more
Colic, 14–15
Colostrum, 35
Comfort items, 243
Common cold. See Coughs, colds, and more
Commonsensemedia.org, 241
Congenital dermal melanocytosis, 191
Congestion, 23–25, 55, 139
Constipation, 96–100. See also Pooping
   frequency of pooping and, 96–97
   fruit juice for, 92
   fruits for, 98, 100
   signs of, 95, 97
   in toddlers, 98–100
Cookie cutters, 84
Cords, loose, 219

Corneal abrasion, 214–215
Coughs, colds, and more,
    135–156. *See also* Fever
    asthma, 149, 156
    breastfeeding mother with,
        53–54
    bronchiolitis treatment,
        151–152
    coughing due to lung infec-
        tion versus pneumonia,
        152–153
    croup, 153–154
    diarrhea with, 101
    ear infections. *See* Ear
        infections
    electrolyte replacement
        solutions for, 70,
        102–103, 115, 116, 129
    green mucus and, 148
    home treatments for cough,
        154–156
    nasal congestion with,
        23–25, 55, 139
    newborn's susceptibility to
        illness, 11, 136
    normal, 137–138
    over-the-counter medicines
        for, 139–140
    pinkeye, 140–141
    respiratory syncytial virus
        (RSV), 150–151
    signs of, 136–137
    sore throat or mouth pain
        with, 145–147
    tips for preventing, 138
    upper respiratory tract
        infections, 148–149
    vaccination during,
        163–164
    wheezing due to, 24,
        148–149, 151
    when to return to child
        care or attend events
        after, 200–201
COVID-19, 137
    vaccine, 11, 165
Cow's milk, 79, 80, 89–90
Cow's milk–based formulas,
    58–59, 67
CPR (cardiopulmonary
    resuscitation), 230
Cracked nipples, 46
Cradle cap, 176–177
Cradle hold, 50
Cribs, 5, 261
Cross-cradle hold, 49, 51
Croup, 153–154
Crying
    in the delivery room,
        2–3
    due to colic, 14–15
    "5 *S*'s" for calming, 15
    pacifiers for, 17–20
    as sign of hunger, 37
    as sign of illness, 15
    swaddling for, 15–17
Cuts and scrapes, 220–221

D

Decongestants, 55
Dehydration
    due to diarrhea, 101–103
    signs of, 104
    when to worry about, 117,
        152
Delivery room, 2–3
Developmental milestones,
    230–235

DHA. *See* Docosahexaenoic acid (DHA)
Diaper bags, 9–10
Diaper cream, 9, 103, 173–175
Diaper rash, 103, 173–175
Diapers, 9
   red streak in, 29–30
   tracking, 71
Diarrhea, 101–106. *See also* Pooping
   after antibiotic, 105–106
   breastfeeding and, 33
   dehydration with, 104
   diaper rash with, 103
   as food allergy symptom, 53, 78
   liquids for treating, 102
   viral causes of, 101
Digital thermometers, 123
Diphtheria, 168
Dislocation, 213–214
Docosahexaenoic acid (DHA), 57, 60
Donor breast milk banks, 34
Doulas, 6, 32, 193, 194
Drapery cords, 219
Dressing your baby, 9, 11–12
Drooling, 130
Drowning, 230
Dysfluencies, 236

E

Ear infections, 141–143
   antibiotic or wait-and-see approach for, 142
   breastfeeding and, 33, 143
   ear tubes and, 143
   middle-ear versus outer-ear, 144
   pacifiers and, 19–20, 143
   risk factors for, 142–143
   when to bathe or swim with, 144–145
Ear pain during air travel, 12–13
Ear tubes, 143
Ear tugging, 141
Eczema, 67, 78, 149, 184–185
Edamame beans, 80
Eggs, 79, 80
   allergies to, 52
   fork-mashed, 77
Electric breast pumps, 41
Electrolyte replacement solutions, 70, 102–103, 115, 116, 129
Elemental formulas, 59
Emergency information, 206
Enfalyte, 70
Erythema toxicum, 175–176
Erythromycin eye ointment, 4
Esophagus, 74
European/Australian formulas, 61
Exercise
   for mothers, 6
   for preventing toilet problems, 99
Eye conditions, 140–141
Eye injuries, 214–215

F

"FaceTiming with Grammie," 240
Facial swelling, 67, 78, 186
Falls, 209–212
Family and Medical Leave Act (FMLA), 194

Fathers, 27, 44, 214
Febrile seizures, 132–133
Feeding and nutrition, 69–92
    allergies and. *See* Food
        allergies
    breast milk. *See*
        Breastfeeding
    burping during, 72
    choking hazards and, 81
    DHA and ARA in, 57, 60
    gas and fussiness after. *See*
        Gas and fussiness
    gastroesophageal reflux
        disease (GERD) and,
        74–75
    infant formula. *See* Bottle-
        feeding
    for mother's milk supply, 45
    organic foods, 60
    picky eaters and, 82–83
    for preventing constipation,
        99
    probiotics in, 39, 57, 60
    toddler formulas, 65
Feeding tube (esophagus), 74
Fenugreek capsules, 45
Fever, 79, 119–133, 147. *See also*
    Coughs, colds, and more
    after vaccines, 119, 131–132,
        160
    alternatives to medicine
        for, 129
    brain damage not caused
        by, 132
    causes of, 120–122
    checking temperature for,
        122–123
    child's behavior as sign of
        less serious, 124

febrile seizure due to,
    132–133
in infant and toddler older
    than 6 months, 122
in infant older than 3
    months, 122
in infant younger than
    3 months, 121, 125,
    131–132, 136–137
medications for, 125–128
with no other symptoms,
    124–125
normal temperature versus,
    120
persisting after fever-
    reducing medications,
    128
with skin infection, 181
sore throat with, 145–147
teething not a cause of, 130
from viruses, 101
Fiber, 99, 100
Fingernails, 22
Firearms, 220
Fire hazards, 219
First aid. *See* Ingestions, inju-
    ries, and first aid
First checkup, 8
Fish, 89
    allergies to, 79, 80
    pureed, 77
"Fish lip" latch, 49
Fish oils, 6
"5 *S*'s," 15
Flat head, 25–26
Fluoride, 64, 227–228
FMLA. *See* Family and Medi-
    cal Leave Act (FMLA)
Folate, 6

Food. *See* Feeding and
    nutrition; Solid foods
Food allergies
    "Big Eight" foods, 79–81
    milk, 58–59, 67, 79, 80,
        88–89
    soy-based formulas and,
        58–59
    spitting up and, 52
    symptoms of, 78–79
Food and Drug Administration
    (FDA), 58, 61, 161
Food colors, 82, 84
Football hold, 49, 51
Foreskin, 28–29
Formula allergy, 67
Formula feeding. *See* Bottle-
    feeding
Forward-facing car seats, 218
Fracture, toddler, 212–213
Fruit juice, 91–92, 100
    watered-down, 91
Fruits, 83, 84
    for constipation, 98, 100

G

Gannon, Polly, 48–49
Gas and fussiness
    bottle-feeding and, 63,
        66–67
    crying due to, 14
    exercises for, 14
    foods that may cause, 53
    mother's diet causing
        baby's, 53
Gastroesophageal reflux
    disease (GERD),
    74–75
Gates, safety, 219

GERD. *See* Gastroesophageal
    reflux disease (GERD)
Glass bottles, 62
Goat milk, 89–90
Goat's rue, 45
Gomco clamp, 27–28
Grapes, 81, 100
Green mucus, 148
Growth and development,
    225–249
    attention-deficit/hyper-
        activity disorder
        (ADHD), 238–239
    autism, 161–162, 237–238
    behavior modification, 244
    developmental milestones,
        230–235
    potty training, 99, 202,
        245–248
    self-soothing skills, 19, 243,
        258–259
    shoes, 228–229
    stuttering, 236
    swimming, 229–230
    talking to baby, 226
    teething, 130, 226–228
    temper tantrums, 241–243
    thumb-sucking, 243
    weight gain, 8, 10, 70–71
Grunting, 153
Guns, 220
Gut bacteria, 15
    bottle-feeding and, 66
    breast milk and, 33

H

Habit reversal training, 243
Haemophilus influenzae type b
    (Hib), 168

Hand, foot, and mouth disease, 146

Hand sanitizer, 9, 138

Handwashing, 13, 138, 201
   after potty use, 248

"Handwashing monitors," 13

Happy spitters, 74

Head control, 50, 75

Head injury, 209–211

Head lice, 187–188

Helmet for reshaping baby's head, 26

Hemangioma, 190

Hemp milk, 89

Hepatitis A, 168

Hepatitis B, 168

Herbal supplements and breastfeeding, 55

Hernias, 112–113

Herpes simplex virus infection, 147

Hib. *See Haemophilus influenzae* type b (Hib)

Hibiclens, 181

Hiccups, 25

Hirschsprung disease, 96

Hives, 67, 78, 88, 186–187

HMO. *See* Human milk oligo-saccharides (HMOs)

Home first-aid kit, 215–216

Honey
   for coughing, 155
   dangers for infants younger than 12 months, 81, 156

Hospital follow-up visit, 10

Hospitalization, 138, 181

Hot dogs, 81

Human milk fortifier, 34

Human milk oligosaccharides (HMOs), 33, 39

Humidifiers, cool-mist, 23, 139, 155

Hunger cues, 37

Hydrocortisone cream, 222

Hypoallergenic formulas, 59

I

Ibuprofen (Motrin or Advil)
   after vaccines, 160
   for air travel, 13
   dosing chart, 127
   for fever, 126–127
   for hand, foot, and mouth disease, 146
   for insect bite or sting, 222
   for pain after falling, 211
   for sore throat or mouth pain, 145

Immune system. *See also* Vaccines
   avoiding crowds due to, 11
   benefits of breastfeeding for, 33
   crying and, 15
   gut bacteria and, 15
   normal, 137–138
   serious illnesses and, 137–138
   viral infections and, 101

Immunizations. *See* Vaccines

Impetigo, 179

Infant formula. *See* Bottle-feeding

Infants (3 months to 1 year)
   amount of sleep needed by, 255
   congestion in, 23–25

developmental milestones in, 232
diarrhea in, 102–103
fever in, 122, 124
head control in, 50, 75
honey dangers for, 81
self-soothing skills in, 19
shoes for, 228–229
signs of readiness for solid food, 75–76
sippy cups for, 84–86
sleep sacks/wearable blanket sleepers for, 17
sunscreen for, 9
talking to, 226
vomiting by, 114–115
water for, 70
Influenza vaccine, 11, 143, 157–158, 164–165, 168
Ingestions, injuries, and first aid, 205–224
  animal bites, 222–223
  babyproofing, 219–220
  car seats and, 216–218
  choking hazards, 81, 208
  coins, 207–208
  emergency information and, 206
  eye injuries, 214–215
  falls and head injury, 209–211
  falls by toddlers, 211–212
  home first-aid kit, 215–216
  insect bite/sting, 221–222
  nursemaid elbow, 213–214
  placing objects up the nose or in the mouth, 208
  splinters, 221
  stitches for cuts, 220–221
  ticks, 223–224
  toddler fracture, 212–213
  what to do after accidental ingestion, 206–207
Inguinal hernias, 112–113
Injuries. *See* Ingestions, injuries, and first aid
Insect bites and stings, 221–222
Iron
  in cereal, 76–77
  supplementation, 39, 57

J

Jaundice, 170–173
Jell-O, 125
Juice. *See* Fruit juice

K

Kale, 89
Kangaroo care. *See* Skin-to-skin contact
Karp, Harvey, 15
K-Y Jelly, 122

L

Lactation consultants, 32, 46, 57
Lactobacillus probiotics, 60
Lactose-free milk, 102
Lactose-free oral rehydration fluids, 102
Laid back hold, 51
La Leche League, 32
Language skills, 226
  milestones, 231–235
  stuttering, 236
Lanolin, 46
Latching, proper, 48–49

Lice, head, 187–188
Liquid concentrate formulas, 61
LiquiLytes, 70
"Loveys," 243
Low-fat (1%) milk, 87
Lyme disease, 223–224

M

Magnesium, 6
Manual breast pumps, 41
Mashed potatoes, 103
Mastitis, 47
Measles, 168
Meat, 77
Meconium, 94
Medications
    acetaminophen. *See*
        Acetaminophen
        (Tylenol)
    antifungal cream, 175
    antihistamine, 55, 187, 222
    anti-itch, 222
    asthma, 149
    avoiding mistakes with, 127
    cantharidin, 182
    cough, 155
    decongestant, 55
    diaper cream, 9, 103,
        173–175
    for fever, 125–128
    ibuprofen. *See* Ibuprofen
        (Motrin or Advil)
    loose stools after antibiotic,
        105–106
    for mastitis, 47
    for methicillin-resistant
        Staphylococcus aureus
        (MRSA), 180–181

for mother feeling over-
    whelmed, 7
for nasal congestion, 55
over-the-counter. *See* Over-
    the-counter medicines
passed through breast milk,
    55
topical antibiotic, 179, 223
Meningitis, 138, 159
Methicillin-resistant *Staphy-
    lococcus aureus* (MRSA),
    180–181
Microwaving
    bottles, 65
    breast milk, 41
Middle-ear infection, 144
Milk alternatives, 89–90
Milk and other liquids
    allergies to, 79, 80, 88–89
    calcium content of, 91
    daily servings of, 90–91
    different types of, 89–90
    filling up on liquid calories, 91
    fruit juice, 91–92, 100
    low-fat (1%) milk, 91
    nondairy milk substitutes,
        88–89
    nonfat milk, 87
    reduced-fat (2%) milk, 87
    sippy cups for, 84–86
    when to introduce regular,
        86–87
    whole milk, 87
Mogen clamp, 28
Molluscum contagiosum,
    181–182
Mothers
    alcohol and caffeine intake
        by, 54–55

baby blues and mood swings in, 6–7

benefits of breastfeeding for, 33

bonding by. *See* Bonding

breast engorgement in, 48

breastfeeding while having a cold, 53–54

breast pain and infection in, 46–47

calling pediatrician for advice. *See* Telephone calls to pediatrician

calories expended while breastfeeding, 33

mastitis in, 47

pumping in the workplace, 43

sleep deprivation in, 7

sore nipples in, 46–47

vaccines for, 157–159

Mother's Milk tea, 45

Motrin. *See* Ibuprofen (Motrin or Advil)

Mouth pain, 145–147

Movement/physical development milestones, 231–235

MRSA. *See* Methicillin-resistant *Staphylococcus aureus* (MRSA)

Mumps, 168

Mupirocin, 179, 181

MyPlate.gov, 84

Myringotomy tubes, 143

N

Nails, 22

Nannies, 195–196

Nasal aspirators, 23, 151, 155

Nasal congestion, 23–25, 55, 139

Nasal saline, 23, 24, 139, 155

Neonatal cephalic pustulosis, 176

Neonatal intensive care unit (NICU), 34–35

Nevus simplex, 189–190

Newborns (0–3 months)

amount of sleep needed by, 255

belly button of, 20–22

bonding with, 3, 4–5

congestion in, 23–25

dehydration in, 117

developmental milestones in, 231

diarrhea in, 102

erythromycin eye ointment for, 4

falls by, 209

feeding schedule of, 37–38

fever in, 121, 123, 125, 131–132, 136–137

first visit with pediatrician, 8

flat head in, 25–26

getting enough to eat, 70–71

immune system in, 11

jaundice in, 170–173

nails of, 22

rashes in, 175–177

sleeping through the night, 252–253

sleep position on back, 5

sleep space for, 5

spitting up by, 52–53, 114

sucking urge in, 18

Newborns (0–3 months)
(*continued*)
sunscreen for, 9
susceptibility to illness, 11,
136
talking to, 226
vaccines for, 158
vitamin K injection in, 3–4
vomiting in, 114
weight loss after birth, 8
*New Mother's Guide to Breast-
feeding*, 32
NICU. *See* Neonatal intensive
care unit (NICU)
Nightlights, 219
Nightmares, 263
Night terrors, 262–263
Nighttime dryness, 248
Nighttime erections, 29
911 calls. *See also* Telephone
calls to pediatrician
accidental ingestion, 207
allergic reactions, 187
breathing trouble, 79
choking, 208
fever, 79
loss of consciousness or
severe injury, 210–211
poisoning, 207
stridor, 79
Nipples
bottle, 63–64
breastfeeding and sore,
46–47
Nipple shells, 46
Nondairy milk substitutes,
88–89
Nonfat milk, 87
Norovirus, 101

Numbing cream, 221
Nursemaid elbow, 213–214
Nursery rhymes, 226
Nurses, baby, 6, 193, 194
Nursing pads, 47
Nursing station, 42
Nutrition. *See* Feeding and
nutrition
Nuts
allergies to, 52
milks, 89
whole, 81

O

Oatmeal, 45, 76, 99
Oat milk, 89
Obstructive sleep apnea,
263–264
Omega-3 fatty acid, 6
Oral rehydration fluids, 70, 102
Oral steroids, 149
Orange juice, 91
Organic formulas, 60
Orthodontic nipples, 63
Otitis externa, 144
Otitis media, 144
Out and about
airplane travel, 12–13
avoiding crowds, 11
baby bag, 9–10
baby carriers/slings for, 5
dressing baby for, 11–12
first pediatrician visit, 8
ordering solid food sides for
baby, 78
premeasuring scoops of
powder formula for
bottle-feeding, 62
Outer-ear infection, 144

Over-the-counter medicines.
    See also Medications
    antihistamines, 55, 187
    anti-itch, 222
    antimicrobial soap, 181
    for colds and coughs,
        139–140
    lice shampoo, 188
    numbing creams, 221
    pinworms, 189
Oxygen treatments, 151

P

Pacifiers, 9
    AAP recommendation on, 18
    for air travel, 13
    ear infections and, 19–20, 143
    interference with breast-
        feeding, 18
    overuse of, 19
    pros/cons of, 17–20
    SIDS and, 17–18
    for soothing, 18
Palivizumab (Synagis), 150
Parents. *See* Fathers; Mothers
PBS Kids, 240
Peanuts, 79, 80
Pea protein milk, 89
Pears, 100
Peas, 75, 99
Pedialyte, 70, 102, 115
Pediatrician. *See also* Tele-
        phone calls to
        pediatrician
    first visit with, 8
    regular visits to, 10
    stomachaches and vomit-
        ing, 110–111
Peppermint tea, 110

Pertussis. *See* Whooping cough
Petroleum jelly, 122
Phototherapy, 173
Pinkeye (conjunctivitis), 140–141
Pinworms, 189
Plagiocephaly, 25–26
Plastibell, 27
Plastic bottles, 62–63
Plug protectors, 219
Plums, 99
Pneumococcus vaccine, 143, 168
Pneumonia, 138, 152–153
    pneumococcus vaccine for,
        143, 168
Poison Control, 206–207
Polio, 168
Pools, 219, 230
Pooping, 71, 93–106. *See also*
        Constipation; Diarrhea;
        Potty training
    appearance of normal poop,
        94–95, 246–247
    frequency of, 96–97
    loose stools after antibiotic,
        105–106
    meconium, 94
Popcorn, 81
Popsicles, 125, 130, 145
Portion sizes, 82–83
Potty chairs, 247
    nighttime dryness and, 248
Potty training, 99. *See also*
        Pooping
    inconsistent success with,
        249
    preschool readiness and, 202
    when to start, 245–246
Powder formulas, 61, 62
Prebiotics, 33, 39

Preschoolers (3–5 years)
  amount of sleep needed by, 256
  readiness for preschool, 202–203
Preterm infants
  breastfeeding of, 34–35
  jaundice in, 171
Probiotics, 39, 57
  in formulas, 60
Projectile vomiting, 114
Protein hydrolysate and elemental formulas, 59
Protein in cow's milk, 90
Prunes, 98, 99, 100
Pumping, breast milk, 40–43
  for child care use, 200
  storage for, 41–42
  when to start, for bottle-feeding, 40–41
  in the workplace, 43
Pureed foods, 75, 77

Q

Quinoa, 76

R

Raisins, 99
Rash
  baby acne, 176
  diaper, 103, 173–175
  erythema toxicum, 175–176
  with fever, 124, 178–179
  roseola, 178–179
  strep throat with, 147
  in toddlers, 177–178
Reading
  to baby, 226
  while sitting on the potty, 247

Ready to feed formulas, 60
Rear-facing car seats, 218
Rectal temperature, 122–123
Red streak in diaper, 29–30
Reduced-fat (2%) milk, 87
Reflux, 73–74, 114. *See also* Spitting up
Respiratory infections and breastfeeding, 33
Respiratory syncytial virus (RSV), 150–151
Retractions, breathing, 24, 152, 153
Reye syndrome, 126
Rice, 103
  brown, 76
Room-temperature formula, 64–65
Rooting, 37
Roseola, 178–179
Rotavirus, 101, 168
Rubella, 168

S

Salmon, 80, 89
Scarlet fever, 147
Scleral icterus, 170
Screen time, 240–241
Seal bark, 153–154
Seborrheic dermatitis, 176–177
Secondhand smoke, 142, 254
Seizures, febrile, 132–133
Self-soothing skills, 19, 243, 258–259
Sesame Street, 240
Shampoos, 176
  for cradle cap, 177
  lice, 188
Sheldon clamp, 27–28

Shellfish, 52, 79
Shoes, 228–229
Siblings, 13
Sick policies, child care,
    197–198, 200–201
Side-lying hold, 51
SIDS. *See* Sudden infant death
    syndrome (SIDS)
Silver nitrate, 21
Singing
    to baby, 226
    while sitting on the potty, 247
Sinus infections, 138
Sippy cups, 84–86
Skin, 169–191
    abscesses, 138
    animal bites, 222–223
    birthmarks, 189–191
    bumps and blemishes on
        newborn, 175–177
    discolored from yellow
        and orange vegetables,
        172–173
    eczema, 67, 78, 149, 184–185
    fever with rash on, 178–179
    head lice, 187–188
    hives, 67, 78, 88, 186–187
    impetigo, 179
    insect bite or sting, 221–222
    jaundice, 170–173
    methicillin-resistant
        Staphylococcus aureus
        (MRSA), 180–181
    molluscum contagiosum,
        181–182
    pinworms, 189
    rash, 103, 124, 177–179
    rash in toddlers, 177–178
    splinters, 221

stitches, 220–221
sunscreen for, 9, 183
ticks on, 223–224
yeast infections, 174, 175
Skin-to-skin contact
    bonding, 3, 5
    delivery room, 3
    for milk production, 34
"Slate-gray" spots. *See* Congeni-
    tal dermal melanocytosis
Sleep, 251–264
    flat head and, 25–26
    improving quality of,
        256–257
    infant/toddler waking up in
        the middle of the night,
        257–259
    mother deprived of, 7
    needed amounts of, 255–256
    newborns sleeping through
        the night, 252–253
    nightmares and night ter-
        rors, 262–263
    nursing baby falling asleep,
        44
    pacifiers for, 18
    placing baby on back for, 5
    snoring, 263–264
    space for newborn, 5, 254
    sudden infant death syn-
        drome (SIDS) and,
        17–18, 33, 254–255
    swaddling for, 15–17
    toddler troubles with,
        259–260
    transitioning from crib to
        big-kid bed for, 261
Sleep apnea, 263–264
Sleep sacks, 17

Smoke and carbon monoxide
    detectors, 219–220
Snoring, 263–264
Social/emotional milestones,
    231–235
Solid foods, 69–92
    "Big Eight" foods, 79–81
    cereal, 76–77
    change in stools with, 94–95
    dozen tries for new, 83
    foods to avoid, 81
    how to introduce, 77–78
    picky eaters and, 82–83
    symptoms of allergies to,
        78–79
    variety of colors of, 84
    when to introduce, 75–76
Sore throat, 145–147
Soy, 79, 80
Soy-based formulas, 58–59
Soy milk, 89
Speech therapy, 236
Sphincter, 74
Spicy foods, 53
Spitting up
    after bottle-feeding, 66–67
    after breastfeeding, 52–53
    causes of, 72–73
    reflux, 73–74, 114
Splinters, 221
Staphylococcus, 179
Stitches, 220–221
Stomachaches and vomiting,
    53, 107–117
    assessing toddlers', 108–109
    bulging belly with, 112–113
    with diarrhea, 102
    due to appendicitis, 111–112
    food allergy, 78

    soothing stomach cramps,
        109–110
    from viruses, 101
    what to give for, 114–116
    when to consult doctor
        about, 110–111
Stomach flu, 101, 110
Stools. *See* Pooping
Storage of expressed breast
    milk, 41–42
Stork bite, 189–190
Strangulation hazards, 219
Strep throat, 147
Streptococcus, 179
Stridor, 79, 153–154
Stuttering, 236
Suctioning, nasal, 23–24
Sudden infant death syndrome
    (SIDS), 17–18
    apnea monitors, 254–255
    breastfeeding and, 33
    room sharing with baby
        and, 254
Sugar water, 70
Sunscreen, 9, 183
Support groups
    breastfeeding, 32
    new-mom, 7
Susceptibility to illness, 11, 136
Swaddling, 15–17
Sweet-tasting drinks, 91–92
Swimmer's ear, 144–145
Swim training, 229–230
Swings, baby, 15
Switching of formulas, 59, 66–67

T

Talking to baby, 226
Tantrums, 241–243

Teeth and teething, 130,
226–228
baby bottle tooth decay, 68
cavities, 228
fluoride for, 64, 227–228
pacifiers and, 19
toothbrushing, 227–228
Telephone calls to pediatrician. *See also* 911 calls
after vaccines, 161, 164
allergic reactions, 187
animal bite, 223
appendicitis, 112
attention-deficit/hyper-
activity disorder
(ADHD), 239
autism, 238
baby not getting enough
colostrum or breast
milk, 36
baby spitting up, 53
baby too sleepy to eat, 44
bacterial skin infection
from bite or sting, 222
breast pain, 47
cold symptoms, 140
concerns after circumci-
sion, 28
constipation, 97
cuts needing stitches,
220–221
decrease in wet and dirty
diapers, 71
dehydration in newborn,
117
developmental milestones,
231
diarrhea, 103
ear pain, 145

feelings of being over-
whelmed or down since
birth, 7
fever, 120–121, 123, 124, 126,
136–137, 147, 164
fever reducers, 128
fever with rash, 179
fever with skin infection,
181
formula allergy, 67
gastroesophageal reflux
disease (GERD), 74–75
head lice, 188
hernia, 113
high-pitched or excessive
crying, 15
infected splinter, 221
jaundice, 173
loose stools, 106
Lyme disease, 224
molluscum contagiosum,
182
newborn feeding schedule,
38
projectile vomiting, 114
rash, 178
redness, swelling, or pain
around penis, 29
red streak in diaper, 30
regarding need for appointment or prescription,
140–141
safety of medications and
herbal supplements,
45
scheduling pediatrician
appointments, 10
seizure, 133
skin infection, 181, 185

Telephone calls to pediatrician. *See also* 911 calls
(*continued*)
sleep concerns, 257
speech therapy referrals,
236
stool color, 95
stopping nursing due to
serious illness, medica-
tion, or treatment, 54
toddler fracture, 213
troubled breathing, 25, 79,
152, 153
umbilical stump, 22
vomiting in older infant or
toddler, 115
wheezing, 149, 152
worries about growth or
weight gain, 83
Television, 240–241
Temperature, checking baby's,
122–123
Temper tantrums, 241–243
Temporal artery (forehead)
thermometers, 123
Tetanus, 168
Thermometers, 122–123
Thimerosal, 162
Thumb-sucking, 243
Ticks, 223–224
Titanium dioxide
sunscreen, 183
Toddler fracture, 212–213
Toddlers (1–3 years)
amount of sleep needed by,
256
animal bites, 222–223
constipation in, 98–100
dairy allergies in, 88–89

developmental milestones
in, 233–235
diarrhea in, 102–103
falls by, 211–212
fever in, 122, 124
formula for, 65
nightmares and night ter-
rors in, 262–263
picky eating habits in,
82–83
portion sizes for, 82–83
potty training of, 99,
245–246
preschool readiness of,
202–203
rash in, 177–178
sleep problems in, 259–260
stomachaches in, 108–109
toddler fracture, 212–213
vitamins for, 81
vomiting by, 114–116
Toenails, 22
Tongue thrust reflex, 75
Tonsils, 264
Topical antibiotics, 179, 223
Toys, 10
as comfort items, 243
Training pants, 248, 249
Transitional milk, 35–36
Tree nuts, 79
Tugging feeling during breastfeeding, 49
Tummy time, 14, 26
for nasal congestion, 24
Tuna, 89
Twins, breastfeeding of, 37
Tylenol. *See* Acetaminophen
(Tylenol)
Tympanostomy tubes, 143

U

Ulcers, mouth, 146–147
Umbilical cord stump, 20–22
Umbilical granuloma, 21–22
Umbilical hernias, 112–113
Upper respiratory tract infections, 148–149
Urate crystals, 29–30

V

Vaccines, 10, 157–166. *See also* Immune system
autism and, 161–162
benefits of, 159
COVID-19, 11, 165
diseases prevented by, 159–160, 168
ear infections and, 143
fever after, 119, 131–132
influenza, 11, 143, 157–158, 164–165, 168
ingredients in, 162–163
for people around baby, 11, 157–159, 164–165
pneumococcus, 143, 168
recommended for children from birth through 6 years old, 167
respiratory syncytial virus (RSV), 150
rotavirus, 101
safety of, 161
schedule for, 163, 167
side effects of, 160–161
when babies have minor illness, 163–164
whooping cough, 157–158
Vegetables, 53, 83, 84
calcium in, 91
fiber in, 99
yellow skin due to yellow and orange, 172–173
Video chatting, 240
Video or computer games, 240–241
Videos, 240–241
Viral infections, 101
croup, 153–154
fever due to, 120
molluscum contagiosum, 181–182
mouth ulcers due to, 146–147
respiratory syncytial virus (RSV), 150–151
roseola, 178–179
sore throat and pink eyes due to, 146
upper respiratory tract infections, 148–149
Vitamin D, 38, 39, 81
Vitamin K injection, 3–4
Vitamins, toddler, 81
Vomiting. *See* Stomachaches and vomiting

W

Washing your hands. *See* Handwashing
Water
for infants older than 6 months, 70
for preventing toilet problems, 99
sterilization for formulas, 64
Watered-down juice, 91
Water heaters, 220

Weight
    diarrhea and loss of, 102
    loss after birth, 8
    regular pediatrician visits
        for checking, 10
    tracking, 70–71
Wharton jelly, 21
Wheat, 79, 80
Wheezing, 24, 148–149
    treatments for, 151–152
Whole-grain foods, 45, 77, 99,
    100
Whole milk, 87
Whooping cough, 11, 159
    vaccine for, 157–158
Window blind cords, 219
Window locks, 219
Wine, 54–55

Withdrawal bleeding, 30
Work, return to
    breast milk pumping and,
        43
    child care options and,
        194–195

Y

Yeast infection, 174, 175
Yogurt, 77, 80
    calcium in, 91
    for constipation, 98

Z

Zinc, 76–77
Zinc oxide
    diaper cream, 103, 173, 175
    sunscreen, 183